Evidence-Based Practice in Nursing

JEAN V. CRAIG, PHD, RSCN, RGN

Jean V. Craig is a research advisor with the Research Design Service of the National Institute of Health Research (NIHR RDS). This varied role entails working with nurses and other healthcare practitioners, methodologists, healthcare managers, and members of the public to develop high-quality, competitive research grant applications.

She has worked as a pediatric nurse in a variety of acute hospitals and settings including the renowned Red Cross War Memorial Children's Hospital, South Africa's only dedicated child health institution, St Thomas' Hospital in London, and Alder Hey Children's Hospital in Liverpool, one of Europe's largest children's hospitals. There, her role as the integrated care pathway coordinator for the cardiac intensive care and other cardiac units provided her with hands-on experience of the challenges of initiating organizational evidence-based practice changes that required buy-in from people from different professions.

Her research career started in Liverpool, where she worked as a research associate in the Evidence-Based Child Health Unit at the University of Liverpool, undertaking systematic reviews and contributing to the development of National clinical guidelines. She was a member of the Alder Hey Children's NHS Trust Research Review Committee and helped to establish and run a Research Clinic at the Trust for clinicians developing research proposals. She established and led the Evidence-Based Practice Child Health module for post-graduates at the University of Liverpool. As a regional research adviser, she has an informal educational role in supporting learning about research methods. She is an independent member of the data monitoring and ethics committees for a number of trials, and a member of the trials adoption group for the Norwich Clinical Trials Unit.

Jean has published on a wide range of nursing topics. She is co-editor of the first three editions of *The Evidence-Based Practice Manual for Nurses*, and is a member of the editorial board for the journal Pilot and Feasibility Studies. Research from her PhD (obtained in Liverpool University, UK) about temperature measurement in infants and children was published in *The Lancet* and the *British Medical Journal*.

DAWN W. DOWDING, PHD, RN, FAAN

Dawn Dowding is Professor in Clinical Decision Making, Division of Nursing, Midwifery and Social Work, School of Health Sciences, University of Manchester, UK. Before this role, she was Professor of Nursing at Columbia University School of Nursing and the Visiting Nurse Service of New York, where she coordinated the Evidence Based Practice module for the nursing curriculum. She is an elected Fellow of the New York Academy of Medicine (NYAM) and the American Academy of Nursing, and was a tutor on the "Teaching Evidence Assimilation for Collaborative Healthcare" (TEACH) program at the NYAM. She is a health services researcher, nurse, and psychologist with expertise in the field of healthcare decision-making and nursing informatics. From 2009 to 2010, she was a Harkness Fellow in Health Care Policy and Practice, working at Kaiser Permanente in Oakland, California. Additional past appointments include Professor of Applied Health Research, University of Leeds UK, and Senior Lecturer in Clinical Decision Making, Hull York Medical School, UK.

She is a member of the editorial board for Worldviews on Evidence-Based Nursing, has published over 90 articles in peer-reviewed journals, and co-authored/co-edited two books on decision-making in nursing.

She completed her registered nurse training at St Bartholomew's College of Nursing and Midwifery, London, has a BSc(Hons) in Psychology with Nursing Studies from City University, London, and a PhD in Psychology and Nursing from the University of Surrey, UK.

FOURTH EDITION

Evidence-Based Practice in Nursing

JEAN V. CRAIG PhD, MSc, RSCN, RGN
Research Advisor, NIHR Research Design Service for the East of England
(Norfolk and Suffolk), Norwich Medical School, University of East Anglia, Norwich, UK

DAWN W. DOWDING PhD, RN, FAAN
Professor in Clinical Decision Making, Division of Nursing, Midwifery and Social Work,
The University of Manchester, Manchester, UK;
Former Professor of Nursing at Columbia University School of Nursing and the Visiting
Nurse Service of New York, New York, USA

ELSEVIER

Edinburgh London New York Oxford Philadelphia St Louis Sydney 2020

ISBN: 978-0-7020-7048-8

Content Strategist: Alison Taylor
Content Development Specialist: Helen Leng, Fiona Conn
Project Manager: Andrew Riley
Design: Brian Salisbury
Marketing Manager: Deborah Watkins

Printed in India

Last digit is the print number: 9 8 7 6 5 4 3

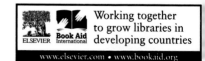

Working together
to grow libraries in
developing countries

www.elsevier.com • www.bookaid.org

CONTENTS

FOREWORD

The shift in healthcare from expert-driven practice to evidence-based healthcare is growing at unprecedented rates. Fueled by educated consumers, spiraling health-care costs and the explosion of information, the demand for evidence-based healthcare has created a situation where one's knowledge of the discipline is often not current or not enough. Former healthcare rituals and traditions that view the practitioner using opinion, experience and pathophysiologic rationale as the primary influencers of practice and clinical decision making are gone. Evidence-based health care is the use of current best evidence in making decisions about the care of individual patients. Best evidence is current, up-to-date, relevant, valid and grounded in research about the effects of a treatment, the potential for harm from exposure to agents, the accuracy of diagnostic tests, and the predictive power of prognostic factors (Cochrane, 1972). Although Archie Cochrane wrote this definition almost 50 years ago, it remains relevant to the practice of evidence-based health care. Point-of-care clinicians and other decision makers need accurate, high quality information to make important decisions.

Nurses challenged by international experts to lead interprofessional healthcare teams in developing and guiding care delivery systems find themselves at the epicenter of this shift—a shift that brings focus to the need for new competencies to affect better patient outcomes. These new competencies include a need to integrate to the extent possible, research, experiential and contextual evidence establishing a culture where evidence is routinely used in daily practice to improve outcomes and increase professional independence. In other words, a practice built on evidence. As such evidence-based practice is a major emphasis in nursing. As a clinical decision-making approach evidence-based practice integrates the best available evidence with experience and the judicious application of this evidence across a variety of patient care situations. This perspective does not challenge individual judgment or the need to incorporate patient values and preferences; rather it puts judgement in the foreground, hugely improved (Holly, Salmond, Saimbert, 2016). Applying and using that evidence in decision making is a critical task. It is, after all, an outcome to which all nurses should strive. The ability to not only understand the literature, but the appraisal, discussion, and application in a sound and thoughtful manner is at the foundation of safe and quality nursing care.

This fourth edition of *Evidence-Based Practice in Nursing* lays the foundation for understanding the importance of an evidence-based approach with a new global perspective that discusses not only the importance of using evidence to guide practice in unique situations, but of understanding how to implement guidelines in specific contexts and the role of Magnet institution status as an influence on evidence-based practice. With online exercises and sample NCLEX questions, this edition explains how to ask the right question, search the literature, evaluate and apply evidence from qualitative, quantitative and mixed methods studies, including systematic reviews. It provides a much-needed perspective on advancing evidence-based practice by explaining how to transform evidence into clinically useful forms, effectively implemented across the entire care experience. Both faculty and students will find it useful in their quest for improved patient outcomes aligned with a practice built on evidence.

Cheryl Holly, RN, EdD, ANEF, FNAP
Professor and Co-Director,
Northeast Institute for Evidence Synthesis and
Translation, a Joanna Briggs Institute
Collaborating Center of Excellence,
Rutgers University School of Nursing,
New Brunswick, New Jersey, USA,
Newark, NJ, USA

References

Cochrane A.(1972). Effectiveness and Efficiency: Random Reflections on Health Services. London: Nuffield Provincial Hospitals Trust. Reprinted in 1989 in association with the *BMJ*. Reprinted in 1999 for Nuffield Trust by the Royal Society of Medicine Press, London.

Holly, C., Salmond, S., Saimbert, M., 2016. Comprehensive Systematic Review for Advanced Nursing Practice. Springer, NY.

"Evidence-based practice" is a concept that has become widespread across health care, and professionals in all clinical practice areas internationally are expected to ensure that their practice is based on evidence. Nurses are the largest group of healthcare professionals and have been at the forefront in recognizing the need to identify, evaluate, and apply best evidence to their clinical practice. Evidence-based practice has now become standard across healthcare environments and is the basis for evaluating quality of care in many healthcare organizations. It is one of the key criteria for a healthcare institution receiving Magnet recognition, a credential awarded to exceptional health care organizations that meet the American Nurses' Credentialing Center (ANCC) standards for quality patient care, nursing, and midwifery excellence and innovations in professional nursing and midwifery practice.

With the acceptance of evidence-based practice in health care have come many advances in the science underlying how to identify, evaluate, and implement evidence into practice. In this fourth edition of the manual, we reflect many of these changes. Most noticeably, this edition includes a new chapter on how to appraise mixed methods studies, and expands the discussion on how to evaluate systematic reviews of qualitative research evidence for quality. It offers a revised discussion of the role of guidelines and their implementation in practice, and includes an updated discussion on the current role of evidence in healthcare organizations. All chapters have been updated. In recognition of the growing international focus on evidence-based practice, we have tried to ensure that the case studies and online exercises that enable readers to consolidate their learning are relevant across different countries.

Nurses, as a profession, remain uniquely placed to understand patients' needs, priorities, and beliefs and to integrate these considerations with their own expertise and with clinical evidence. The result of these endeavors is that better clinical decisions will be made and patient care will improve.

Jean V. Craig ■ *Dawn W. Dowding*

The editor(s) would like to acknowledge and offer grateful thanks for the input of all previous editions' contributors, without whom this new edition would not have been possible.

Olwen Beaven, BSc (Hons), MSc
Information Specialist, BMJ Knowledge Centre, BMJ, London, UK

Diane Bunn, PhD, MSc, BSc (Hons)
Lecturer in Nursing Sciences (Adult), School of Health Sciences, University of East Anglia, Norwich, UK

Bernie Carter, PhD
Professor of Children's Nursing, Faculty of Health and Social Care, Edge Hill University, Ormskirk, Lancashire, UK

Jean V. Craig, PhD, MSc, RSCN, RGN
Research Advisor, NIHR Research Design Service for the East of England (Norfolk and Suffolk), Norwich Medical School, University of East Anglia, Norwich, UK

Dawn W. Dowding, PhD
Professor in Clinical Decision Making, Division of Nursing, Midwifery and Social Work, University of Manchester, Manchester, UK

Helena Dunbar, PhD, MSc, BA (Hons)
Interim Associate Professor Maternal and Child Health, Leicester School of Nursing and Midwifery, De Montfort University, Leicester, UK

Kate Flemming, PhD, MSc, PG Cert, BSc (Hons)
Senior Lecturer, Health Sciences, University of York, York, UK

Sarah Hanson, RGN, MA, PhD
Lecturer in Nursing Science, University of East Anglia, Norwich, UK

Leanne V. Jones, BSc, MMedSci
Associate Editor, Cochrane Pregnancy and Childbirth Group, Department of Women's and Children's Health, Institute of Translational Medicine, University of Liverpool, Liverpool, UK

Gillian A. Lancaster, PhD, MSc, BSc (Hons)
Professor, Institute of Primary Care and Health Sciences, Keele University, Keele, UK

Gareth McCray, PhD MRes, MA, BA (Hons)
Research Associate, Keele University, Keele, UK

Patricia Quinlan, PhD, MPA
Assistant Vice President Nursing Excellence, Dawn Dowling School of Nursing, Columbia University, New York, USA

Arlene Smaldone, PhD, RN
Professor of Nursing, Columbia University School of Nursing, New York, USA, Professor of Dental Behavioral Sciences, College of Dental Medicine, Columbia University, New York, USA; Assistant Dean, Scholarship and Research, Columbia University School of Nursing, New York, USA

Carl Thompson, PhD
Professor, School of Healthcare, University of Leeds, Leeds, UK

CHAPTER 1

Evidence-Based Practice in Nursing

Jean V. Craig ■ Dawn W. Dowding

KEY POINTS

- An evidence-based approach to clinical practice aims to deliver appropriate care in an efficient manner to individual patients so that the optimum outcome can be achieved.
- Policies have helped to drive forward the evidence-based practice (EBP) movement, changing the face of nursing education.
- The process for EBP entails the integration of research evidence, clinical expertise, and the interpretation of patients' needs and perspectives in making decisions. It starts with converting information needs about clinical problems into clear questions, seeking evidence to answer those questions, and then evaluating (critically appraising) the evidence for its validity (truthfulness) and usefulness.
- Much has been done to facilitate this process. For example, evidence has been synthesized in high-quality systematic reviews, clinical guidelines have been developed, and there are computerized decisions support systems to offer point-of-care guidance. However, a number of challenges remain.
- It is the responsibility of the individual nurse to develop the key skills and key competencies required to access and use evidence appropriately in clinical practice.
- Organizational culture plays a crucial part in determining the extent to which EBP is pursued by healthcare practitioners; support from management, training to ensure relevant professional development, provision of high-quality evidence at point of care, empowering nurses, teamwork, and shared decision-making all play a role.
- A number of models or frameworks have been published that offer important perspectives on embedding an evidence-based approach to care within the organization.

Evidence-Based Health Care: What Is It and Why Do We Need It?

Evidence-based practice (EBP) has been defined as "a problem-solving approach to the delivery of health care that integrates best evidence from studies and patient care data with clinician expertise and patient preferences and values" (Melnyk et al., 2010). It has also previously been described as doing the right things right (Muir Gray, 1997, p. 18) so, not only doing things efficiently and to the best standard possible, but also ensuring that that which is done is of known effectiveness for that clinical situation, resulting in more good than harm. The point here is that, if we can get it right, EBP will help to improve people's experiences of illness and health care. Intuitively, few practitioners would disagree with this approach, but there are several hurdles on the way to this goal: we need the evidence base to know what it is "right" to do (and evidence generally lags behind practice), we have to be clear to whom the evidence really applies and at what stage in their trajectory of health or illness an evidence-based intervention is indicated, and we need to implement that intervention efficiently.

USING EVIDENCE TO INFORM PRACTICE: A LONG ESTABLISHED CONVENTION

The concept of EBP is certainly not new. We would be doing our predecessors a great disservice to pretend otherwise. Let us take the example of infection control, a long-established aspect of nursing care that aims to prevent complications arising from vulnerability to infection. Semmelweis' observations on puerperal fever in the 1840s led to him insisting that doctors performing autopsies should wash their hands before going on to deliver babies, and this was associated with a marked reduction in mortality due to sepsis from over one-fifth to 3% (Rotter, 1997). Similarly, it was careful observation that led John Snow in the 1840s to pinpoint a water tap in Broad Street as the cause of the outbreak of cholera in London. These examples from the 19th century encapsulate the variety of domains of professional health practice that can and should be evidence based, but they also demonstrate powerfully how reflective questioning and acutely observant practitioners can uncover evidence within their own everyday practice, which, when acted on, can improve health, although not all examples will be quite so dramatic!

It is perhaps cruelly ironic given the examples mentioned earlier that, in an era in which EBP is generally considered a key component of modern health care, patients are at continued risk of developing healthcare-associated infections (HAIs). HAI prevalence, although decreasing, has been estimated at 4% (95% CI, 3.7–4.4) among hospitalized patients in the US (Magill et al., 2014). Approximately 440,000 adult inpatients a year suffer HAIs, commonly surgical site and *Clostridium difficile* infections (Zimlichman et al., 2013). Across Europe, the estimated mean prevalence for HAI is 6% (country range 2.3%–10.8%) (European Centre for Disease Prevention and Control, 2013) with approximately 24% of those infections being pneumonia or lower respiratory tract infections, 20% surgical site infections, and 19% urinary tract infections.

Costs attributable to HAIs are considerable from both hospital and societal perspectives; morbidity, mortality, increased length of hospital stay, and financial costs to healthcare providers and patients and families are substantial. In the US adult population alone, the estimated annual cost of five major HAIs (surgical site infection, central line–associated bloodstream infection, catheter-associated urinary tract infection, ventilator-associated pneumonia, and *Clostridium difficile* infection) are $9.8 billion, with over one-third of the cost attributed to surgical site infections (Zimlichman et al., 2013). HAIs are especially worrying in view of the risk of antibiotic-resistant infections such as methicillin-resistant *Staphylococcus aureus*.

Reasons for HAIs are multiple: patient factors (e.g., increased numbers of people with weakened immunity), therapeutic factors (increased availability of devices that breach normal defense mechanisms and inappropriate use of antibiotics), behavioral factors (inadequate hygiene practices by staff, carers, visitors, and patients), and organizational factors (e.g., increased movement of patients) are all cited (Department of Health, 2003; Castro-Sánchez and Holmes, 2015). A significant proportion of HAIs are preventable; recent systematic reviews have indicated that organizations with a positive patient safety climate lead to greater adherence to standard precautions for infection control (Hessels and Larson, 2016) and that some combinations of quality improvement interventions (e.g., education, audit and feedback, reminder systems, and organizational change) can improve adherence to infection-control practices and reduce infection rates (Mauger et al., 2014). Although both reviews highlighted that there are issues with the quality of evidence in this area, and heterogeneity in how studies are conducted, what this does indicate is that implementing practices that are informed by scientific evidence, where available, can help improve outcomes for patients. Tools such as those produced by the Centers for Disease Control and Prevention in the US have been developed to assist health facilities (acute care, long-term, hemodialysis, and outpatient care facilities) in assessing their infection-prevention practices and making quality improvements (https://www.cdc.gov/hai/prevent/infection-control-assessment-tools.html).

THE EVIDENCE-BASED MOVEMENT ACROSS HEALTH CARE

In the early years of the evidence-based "movement," the discourse was limited to "medicine," rather than health care (Sackett et al., 1997), but the principles of evidence-based medicine have subsequently been applied to other spheres of professional practice in health and social care, such as pharmacy (Eriksson et al., 2014), the therapies (Scurlock-Evans et al., 2014; Upton et al, 2014), and orthodontics (Madhavji et al., 2011). Nursing has fully embraced EBP as a strategy for providing the highest quality of care, with key professional organizations such as the American Association of Colleges of Nursing (AACN) developing curricula to incorporate elements of EBP, and the role of implementation of EBP in Magnet hospital recognition (Correa-de-Araujo, 2016).

In 2000, the Institute of Medicine (IOM) published *To Err Is Human,* which reported the prevalence of deaths and injury occurring from healthcare errors (IOM, 2000). As a result of this publication, attention to quality and safety peaked, and other widespread defects in the US healthcare system were also identified (IOM, 2001). Quickly following these reports, recommendations were made in the *Quality Chasm* series that underscored the centrality of EBP as a solution in redesigning care that is effective and safe (IOM 2001, 2003, 2008). The EBP movement was significantly accelerated by these reports, and key recommendations were made: (i) to provide services based on scientific knowledge to all who could benefit (IOM, 2001), (ii) to educate all healthcare professionals to deliver evidence-based care (IOM, 2003), and (iii) to assess the effectiveness of clinical services to provide unbiased information about what really works in health care (IOM, 2008). Nurse experts echoed these recommendations: employing EBP was a competency expected of nurses (Stevens and Staley, 2006).

In the UK, following a review of the National Health Service (NHS) led by health minister and surgeon Lord Darzi, there was a shift in health policy. Whereas the emphasis had been on reducing waiting times, ensuring faster access to care, and giving more choice to patients, a broader view on quality—defined as patient safety, patient experience, and effectiveness of care—dictated policy (Department of Health, 2008). Alongside key initiatives such as the introduction of comparable quality indicators and the publishing of patient-reported/clinical outcomes to allow practitioners to benchmark their own performance against that of others, an improved information resource was introduced to aid the delivery of effective care. *NHS evidence* is a web-based portal giving practitioners easy access to "authoritative clinical and non-clinical evidence and best practice" required for effective clinical decision-making. It is considered by Lord Darzi as an essential service that allows quality to be "stitched into the very fabric of the NHS" (Department of Health, 2009). The code of conduct for nurses and midwives implemented in March 2015, and updated in October 2018, served to further embed this notion of evidence driving quality, with the standard for effective practice explicitly mentioning the role of evidence: "You assess need, and deliver or advise on treatment, or give help (including preventative or rehabilitative care) without too much delay, to the best of your abilities, on the basis of best available evidence" (Nursing and Midwifery Council, 2018, p. 9).

One needs only to look at the Standards of Nursing Practice or Codes of Conduct developed in countries such as Canada, Australia, and New Zealand (Nursing Midwifery Council, 2018) (Canadian Nurses Association, 2017; Nursing and Midwifery Board of Australia, 2016; Nursing Council of New Zealand, 2012) to appreciate that EBP has international traction.

WHAT DOES IT LOOK LIKE IN PRACTICE?

The first textbook on evidence-based medicine (EBM) defined it as: "the conscientious, explicit and judicious use of current best evidence in making decisions about the health care of patients" (Sackett et al., 1997, p. 2). The authors elaborated that the practice of EBM entailed the integration of individual clinical expertise with the best available external clinical evidence from systematic research, and it involved taking account of the patient's perspective in making clinical decisions. Contrary to the assertions of its early critics, therefore, that EBM was narrowly concerned with the conduct of randomized controlled trials and the implementation of their results in routine practice (Grahame Smith, 1998), the product champions of EBM never argued that it was "simply" a matter of slavishly following rigid guidelines based solely on the findings of trials; the need to tailor care on the basis of research evidence and clinical experience to the needs of patients was always acknowledged.

In 2000, Sackett et al. included the value of clinical expertise and patient perspectives more explicitly in their definition of EBM as "the integration of best research evidence with clinical expertise and patient values" (Sackett et al., 2000, p. 1). They define their terms carefully. Best research evidence is defined as:

clinically relevant research, often from the basic sciences of medicine (sic), but especially from patient-centered clinical research…

SACKETT ET AL., 2000, P. 1

They go on to assert that:

New evidence from clinical research both invalidates previously accepted diagnostic tests and treatments and replaces them with new ones that are more powerful, more accurate, more efficacious and safer

SACKETT ET AL., 2000, P. 1

Note that the discourse is about "diagnostic tests" and "treatments," whereas the broader concept of "care," which embodies nursing practice in all settings, involves much more, such as communication and observation. This means that, in applying these principles to the variety of nursing practice, we need to draw on a range of evidence bases including from psychology and sociology.

Clinical expertise is defined as:

the ability to use our clinical skills and past experience to rapidly identify each patient's unique health state and diagnosis, their individual risks and benefits of potential interventions, and their personal values and expectations

SACKETT ET AL., 2000, P. 1

Personal professional experience, clinical judgment, and even intuition have a role to play. By "*patient values*," the authors mean:

the unique preferences, concerns and expectations each patient brings to a clinical encounter and which must be integrated into clinical decisions if they are to serve the patient

SACKETT ET AL., 2000, P. 1

In reality, then, EBP is manifest by the integration of systematically derived research-based knowledge with the practitioner's tacit knowledge drawn from experience and their interpretation of the needs and perspectives of each person with whom they interact in individual clinical encounters.

The steps in the EBP process entail:
1. converting information needs about clinical problems into clear questions
2. seeking evidence to answer those questions
3. evaluating (critically appraising) the evidence for its validity (truthfulness) and usefulness
4. integrating findings with clinical expertise, patient needs, and patient preferences to reach a decision as to the optimum course of action, and then applying this decision
5. evaluating performance and the outcome of the decision.

The principles enunciated by Sackett et al. are clearly of direct relevance to all professional practice, but for any practitioner this is a daunting agenda. In the early days of EBP, we believed it meant that each individual clinician should access, appraise, and synthesize evidence from primary research studies to develop guidelines. Today, the move is toward research knowledge being transformed into clinical recommendations by expert panels, and embedded into healthcare delivery systems in the form of, for example, electronic prompts or reminders. Technological developments have led to the increasing use of computerized decision support systems, which have been defined as: "information systems aimed to support clinical decision-making, linking patient-specific information in electronic health records with evidence-based knowledge to generate case-specific guidance messages through a rule- or algorithm-based software" (Moja et al., 2014). That said, it remains imperative that practitioners learn to be wise users of the different types and forms of evidence integral to good patient care and to know which evidence is informative in selecting actions that have the highest likelihood of producing the intended patient outcome.

Workforce Competencies for Evidence-Based Practice

The new competencies that emerged with the EBP movement require healthcare professionals to engage in knowledge (evidence) management—to access knowledge, to appraise knowledge, and to integrate new knowledge into practice changes. Continued professional development for lifelong learning has long been recognized as essential to quality care (Department of Health, 2001; IOM, 2001) and for more than a decade, EBP competencies have been articulated across health professions (IOM, 2003).

Specifically in nursing, EBP competencies were developed from several perspectives. In the US, following the recommendations that each health profession must develop its specific competencies, national consensus was established across a set of 82 competency statements; the competencies were organized around the five points of the ACE Star Model of Knowledge Transformation (Stevens, 2004) discussed later in this chapter (discovery, summary, translation, integration, and evaluation), and across three levels of professional preparation (basic, intermediate, and advanced). These competencies guide the retooling of current workforce and the preparation (education) of future workforce. They form the foundation for the ACE Evidence-Based Practice Readiness Inventory, a survey of self-efficacy in employing EBP (Stevens, 2009; Stevens et al., 2009).

After these developments, a widespread effort emerged to support the identification of competencies for quality and safety education in nursing (Cronenwett et al., 2007). Within this ongoing project, national panels are engaged in identifying competencies in EBP, patient-centered care, teamwork and collaboration, quality improvement, safety, and informatics, reflecting the recommendations from the IOM (2003). To assist with the full adoption into educational programs, the Quality and Safety Education for Nurses program includes significant teaching-learning resources on the website (QSEN, 2010). Specific EBP competencies are now included as essential competencies for baccalaureate, masters, and doctoral education in the US (AACN, 2006, 2008, 2011). More recently, Melnyk et al. (2014) developed a set of competencies for registered nurses (RN) and advanced practice nurses (APNs) in the US, using consensus methods. The set consists of 13 competencies for practicing RNs and a further 11 competencies for APNs.

A Wide Range of Evidence Bases Relevant to Nursing Practice

In making decisions about therapies, investigations, service provision, and so on, nurses need to draw on a wide range of evidence sources within and beyond the "medical" sciences, as illustrated in our earlier discussion of healthcare-associated infections and in the examples that follow.

Concordance or adherence with drug therapy can be influenced by various factors including social and economic factors (e.g., level of social support, living environment, cost of drugs); the relationship between the patient and provider; the nature of the illness (with concordance a challenge for chronic illnesses treated over a long period); the medications themselves (e.g., the number of medications, number of daily doses, side effects); and patient factors (e.g., cognitive impairment, lack of knowledge, substance abuse) (Kalogianni, 2011; Mathes et al., 2014; Vangeli et al., 2015). The approach to the problem of poor concordance with treatment therefore requires knowledge from the psychosocial and pharmacological domains.

Nurses wanting to introduce costly services such as a new clinic or nursing post will increasingly be obliged to present to the management team evidence on not only the effectiveness and potential harms of the intervention, but also the cost-effectiveness.

In management sciences, the research task is often to understand the organization and how change is perceived, as much as to study the effectiveness of a complex process of change, and nurses can draw on a wide range of quantitative and qualitative research to help them become more effective managers. In the US, the Agency for Healthcare Research and Quality conducts research into the healthcare delivery system and provides tools (e.g., materials for teaching and training healthcare professionals), with the goal of making the healthcare system safer and implementing research into practice. In the UK, the National Institute of Health Research has a Health Services and Delivery Research program focused on producing evidence to improve the quality, accessibility, and organization of health and social care services.

For effective communication with communities, clients, and patients, nurses can draw on communication studies and psychology. Psychological research has shown that on receiving bad news, recipients retain only a limited amount of information from the first conversation; nurses can use these findings when imparting bad news, by keeping their first message simple, and providing ongoing support and repeated conversations to enable information to be given at a pace with which recipients can cope.

Nurses working in public health roles may be in a key position to advocate initiatives supported by evidence from research in the public health domain. A notable public health example is the introduction of legislation to make the wearing of seatbelts compulsory, based on epidemiological evidence of reductions in mortality.

TYPES OF EVIDENCE

When thinking about the different evidence bases, it is also worth considering the "types of evidence" that can guide practice. Evidence-based clinical guidelines play a key role in EBP. They comprise sets of recommendations for clinical practice that have been systematically developed by a guideline development group following careful consideration of the available evidence. Ideally, that evidence would comprise a body of well-conducted scientific research studies. However, often there are no such studies available, and other sources of evidence such as data from audits, service evaluation, or other sources may be the best available data. Table 1.1 gives a helpful overview of the differences between research, audit, and service evaluation, produced by the NHS Health Research Authority (2017).

TABLE 1.1 ■ Research, Service Evaluation and Audit Compared

Research	Service Evaluation	Clinical/ Non-Financial Audit	Usual Practice (in Public Health Including Health Protection)
The attempt to derive generalizable or transferable new knowledge to answer questions with scientifically sound methods* including studies that aim to generate hypotheses as well as studies that aim to test them, in addition to simply descriptive studies.	Designed and conducted solely to define or judge current care.	Designed and conducted to produce information to inform delivery of best care.	Designed to investigate the health issues in a population in order to improve population health. Designed to investigate an outbreak or incident to help in disease control and prevention.
Quantitative research—can be designed to test a hypothesis as in a randomized controlled trial or can simply be descriptive as in a postal survey. Qualitative research—can be used to generate a hypothesis, usually identifies/explores themes.	Designed to answer: "What standard does this service achieve?"	Designed to answer: "Does this service reach a predetermined standard?"	Designed to answer: "What are the health issues in this population and how do we address them?" Designed to answer: "What is the cause of this outbreak or incident and how do we manage it?"
Quantitative research—addresses clearly defined questions, aims and objectives. Qualitative research—usually has clear aims and objectives but may not establish the exact questions to be asked until research is underway.	Measures current service without reference to a standard.	Measures against a standard.	Systematic, quantitative or qualitative methods may be used.
Quantitative research—may involve evaluating or comparing interventions, particularly new ones. However, some quantitative research such as descriptive surveys, do not involve interventions. Qualitative research—seeks to understand better the perceptions and reasoning of people.	Involves an intervention in use only. The choice of treatment, care or services is that of the care professional and patient/service user according to guidance, professional standards and/or patient/service user preference.	Involves an intervention in use only. The choice of treatment, care or services is that of the care professional and patient/service user according to guidance, professional standards and/or patient/service user preference.	Involves an intervention in use only. Any choice of intervention, treatment, care or services is based on best public health evidence or professional consensus.

Continued

TABLE 1.1 ■ Research, Service Evaluation and Audit Compared—cont'd

Research	Service Evaluation	Clinical/ Non-Financial Audit	Usual Practice (in Public Health Including Health Protection)
Usually involves collecting data that are additional to those for routine care but may include data collected routinely. May involve treatments, samples or investigations additional to routine care. May involve data collected from interviews, focus groups and/or observation.	Usually involves analysis of existing data but may also include administration of interview(s) or questionnaire(s).	Usually involves analysis of existing data but may include administration of simple interview or questionnaire.	May involve analysis of existing routine data supplied under license/agreement or administration of interview or questionnaire to those in the population of interest. May also require evidence review.
Quantitative research—study design may involve allocating patients/service users/healthy volunteers to an intervention. Qualitative research—does not usually involve allocating participants to an intervention.	No allocation to intervention: the care professional and patient/service user have chosen intervention before service evaluation.	No allocation to intervention: the care professional and patient/service user have chosen intervention before audit.	No allocation to intervention.
May involve randomization.	No randomization.	No randomization.	May involve randomization but not for treatment/care/intervention.
Normally requires REC review but not always. Refer to http://hra-decisiontools.org.uk/ethics/ for more information.	Does not require REC review.	Does not require REC review.	Does not require REC review.

*UK Policy Framework for Health and Social Care Research definition of research (full details available from HRA website)
NHS Health Research Authority October 2017. Defining Research. Copyright & other intellectual property rights in this material belong to the Health Research Authority: www.hra.nhs.uk. With permission.

Challenges

The challenge, then, for clinical nursing practice is to utilize the well-focused evidence base relating to specific clinical treatments to improve the quality of clinical procedures, while also drawing on a more diverse evidence base for the wider concept of care that nurses provide. This challenge is not straightforward, and there are several imperatives to be addressed.

GAPS IN EVIDENCE

First, the relevant research-based evidence bases are not comprehensive. Historically, academic and clinical nursing existed as two separate entities, resulting in much research being unrelated to the "reality" of everyday nursing practice (Pearson, 2000). This historical trend in research, of prioritizing professional issues over patient care issues, had important ramifications for nurses trying to make informed decisions about aspects of clinical care. Happily this situation has changed dramatically, with clinically relevant research burgeoning. Although, of course, there remain gaps in the robust evidence for much of what nurses (and other healthcare professionals) do in the course of their daily work.

It is important that the recognition of the need for evidence does not result in a misguided and undiscerning dash to seek out *any "knowledge"* available, irrespective of the quality of research on which it is based. Critical appraisal skills are crucial to enable practitioners who are thirsty for knowledge to discriminate between high- and low-quality evidence: to be cognizant of the strengths and weaknesses of the various research methodologies used to generate different kinds of evidence, to assess for rigor of the study design and conduct, and to be clear about to whom the research applies. Where there is no robust evidence base, the ethos of EBP should stop us in our tracks to reflect on the impact of what we are doing in the name of health, and why. Reflective practice is a key component of evidence-based health care; the very ethos of good professional practice is to reflect on the taken-for-granted assumptions that underpin everyday practice and to routinely assess the impact and outcomes of interactions and interventions with patients, clients, and the public. And we need to do all this without becoming "frozen" and disempowered by a paucity of robust evidence.

TOO MUCH EVIDENCE

Having pointed out the challenge of a lack of evidence, in some areas of health care there has been a great deal of research, and it is almost impossible for any busy practitioner to keep abreast of the burgeoning body of information that emerges daily. Furthermore, the results and conclusions of one study need to be considered in the light of other similar studies as they may differ markedly, depending on the nature of the study design and sample. An oft-quoted example is that of corticosteroids given to women expected to deliver prematurely. A number of trials did not identify clear-cut benefits of the treatment; however, when data from all trials included in a systematic review were combined in a meta-analysis, it became clear that corticosteroids are effective in reducing the risk of death in babies born prematurely (Mulrow, 1995). Today, systematic reviews are widely endorsed as an authoritative basis for informing practice decisions by weighty organizations such as the National Institute for Health and Clinical Excellence (2012). Indeed the Institute of Medicine (US) Committee on Standards for Developing Trustworthy Clinical Practice Guidelines (2011) asserts that "The idea that trustworthy clinical practice guidelines should be based on a high-quality SR (systematic review) of the evidence is beyond dispute."

Added to this challenge of "too much evidence," clinical problems need to be examined from various perspectives. If an emphasis is placed solely on determining the effectiveness of an intervention on say one narrow outcome, an oversimplified and unbalanced decision may be reached.

Consideration of evidence that investigates a broader range of outcomes and patients' past experiences of the intervention could well lead to a different, more informed decision. It is hardly surprising that accessibility to just the right information (no less, no more) is flagged as an important facilitator for the adoption of an evidence-based approach to health care (Campbell et al., 2015; Veeramah, 2016).

We need effective means by which robust evidence is integrated with the existing knowledge base in a timely manner, and made available to practitioners at time of need, in a readily accessible format. Greenhalgh et al. (2014) call for producers of evidence-based materials and clinical decision support tools to be cognizant of not only the end user, but also the purpose for which the materials and tools will be used and the constraints within which they will be used. Perhaps as a way of encouraging this development, they entreat patients to demand evidence that is better, better presented, and better explained.

EVIDENCE MAY NOT BE APPLICABLE TO A SPECIFIC CLINICAL SETTING OR PATIENT GROUP

Third, research findings should not always be transferred directly into the clinical setting. It is crucial that evidence from studies undertaken with a specific population is not inappropriately and unthinkingly extrapolated to other population subgroups, such as to patients of a different age group. Clinical trials in people over 80 years of age are scarce (Shenoy and Harugeri, 2015), with the majority of trials being undertaken in samples of people under the age of 65. Care should be taken if extrapolating research findings from such trials to older people who could have several coexisting conditions or other unique risk factors that may prevent them from attaining the same results as those attained by the (younger) trial participants.

Healthcare organizations and individuals are responsible for ascertaining whether or not evidence is likely to be generalizable to their patient populations, and if so, to adapt or localize practice recommendations before piloting then implementing them and evaluating their effect.

THE ORGANIZATION MAY NOT FOSTER A CULTURE OF EVIDENCE-BASED PRACTICE

This leads to a final point, the challenge for the organization to develop and maintain a supportive culture, which provides a foundation for the delivery of high-quality care that can improve the lives of patients and their carers, through team working and shared decision. Nurses need to be autonomous and empowered through, for example, being given opportunities for learning and professional progression (Echevarria et al., 2017). In their thought-provoking paper entitled "Evidence based medicine: a movement in crisis," Greenhalgh et al. (2014) point out the risk of a gradual slide toward the misuse of evidence, where algorithmic rules and prompts lead to a technocratic approach to care, in which patients are sent for tests or started on therapies without being offered personalized shared decision-making and individualized care. Organizations therefore need a culture of supporting training and development so that health care practitioners are not just able to find and critically read research evidence, but are also able to apply their expert judgment and to have meaningful conversations with patients when reaching clinical decisions about care; the practitioner-patient relationship needs to be foremost if the founding principles of EBP are to be followed (Greenhalgh et al., 2014).

Frameworks for Evidence-Based Practice

The most elemental concept in engaging practitioners in EBP is the *form* of knowledge (evidence) to which they connect. As already discussed, knowledge should be presented in a form that has high utility to clinical decision-making. Rather than requiring practitioners to master the technical expertise to critique scientific adequacy of a primary research study, their point-of-care decisions would be much better supported with recommendations that have been based on all existing research knowledge and vetted by clinical experts.

A number of models (some described as frameworks or guidelines) have been published that offer important perspectives on embedding an evidence-based approach to care within the organization, as discussed by Schaffer et al. (2013). We present just two models in the following section as examples, but see Schaffer et al. (2013) for a useful summary of these and four additional models: Advancing Research and Clinical Practice Through Close Collaboration (ARCC); the Johns Hopkins Nursing Evidence-Based Practice Model (JHNEBP); Promoting Action on Research Implementation in Health Services Framework (PARIHS); the Stetler Model.

The IOWA model was developed and further revised by Titler et al. (2001) and has subsequently been further updated by the Iowa Model Collaborative (2017) in collaboration with stakeholders. Reasons given for the update include widespread use of electronic data; enhanced patient engagement; the upsurge in synthesized evidence; the emergence of implementation science, defined as "the scientific study of methods to promote the systematic uptake of research findings and other EB practices into routine practice healthcare...to improve the quality and effectiveness of health services and care" (Eccles and Mittman, 2006); and associated initiatives promoting uptake of EBP.

The first step in the model is to identify triggering problems or opportunities that arise in the course of clinical practice or as a result of new data, new evidence, new initiatives, or regulations. This "trigger" generates a question. The next step is to reach a decision on whether the topic is a priority for the organization. If so, a team of stakeholders is assembled, with the required skills. They search for, critique, and synthesize the available body of evidence (weighing the quality, quantity, consistency, and risk of the evidence). If the evidence base is lacking, this flags an opportunity for future research. However, if the evidence is deemed sufficient to affect a change in practice, and the change is considered appropriate, the next step is to design a practice change that will fit the unique setting in which it is to be applied. This is done in collaboration with patients and carers to incorporate their preferences and values, while taking account of resources and other organizational constraints and preferences. An implementation plan and related materials are developed and promoted, and staff are prepared for the change. A pilot of the change follows, with collection of baseline and follow-up data that are examined to determine whether it is indeed appropriate to adopt the change as designed. If yes, and adopted, then ongoing work is taken to sustain the change. This includes ongoing monitoring, engaging key personnel who can drive and champion the change, and "hardwiring" the change into the system so that it is automatically facilitated.

The ACE Star Model of Knowledge Transformation (Stevens, 2004) provides a framework with which to consider the transformation of knowledge from its point of discovery to its impact on patient and healthcare outcomes. Depicted as a five-point star to indicate the various stages of knowledge transformation, the model is conceptualized as follows: (i) Discovery: undertaking primary research. (ii) Evidence summary: synthesizing the evidence from primary research studies, ideally using rigorous systematic review methodology. (iii) Translation: developing EBP guidelines; a process in which experts consider the evidential base, combine it with expertise and theory, and extend recommendations for practice. (iv) Integration: practice is aligned or realigned to reflect best evidence and is tailored to the particular healthcare setting and patient-centered preferences. (v) Evaluation: taking an inclusive view of the impact that the EBP has on patient health outcomes, satisfaction, efficacy, and efficiency of care and health policy. Quality improvement of healthcare processes and outcomes is the goal of knowledge transformation. A preferred starting point in moving evidence into clinical decisions is point 3: finding clinical recommendations that are clearly evidence based. Once this is accomplished, the clinician considers point 4, integration into practice, and adopts the recommendations into local practice.

Models allow us to conceptualize the process of "operationalizing" EBP. They can contribute to our understanding of how to change practice in the light of best evidence within the context of knowledge translation/implementation science. Considerable research of implementation has been conducted using theoretical approaches, which can be helpful in terms of informing approaches to implementation (Nilsen, 2015), but there remain gaps in our knowledge, with a call for a broader research agenda that encompasses "the psychology of evidence interpretation" and "the negotiation and sharing of evidence by clinicians and patients" (Greenhalgh et al., 2014).

It is worth noting that there is still much to learn about which methods, or combinations of methods, are most useful in helping individuals to adopt an evidence-based approach in their day-to-day practice. Further information about the effectiveness of behavior change interventions such as seminars, conferences, audit with feedback, real-time reminders, and clinical guidelines is provided in Chapter 10.

Conclusion

Nursing education has been transformed in response to the EBP movement. The current workforce, new workforce, and future workforce are essential in successfully ensuring a paradigm of care that fully employs EBP. Education, professional development, performance expectations, managers, organizational leaders, and policy makers are powerful factors in achieving this change.

The following chapters in this manual are designed to further develop your skills for competence in EBP—not just your skills in focusing your clinical questions (Chapter 2); finding research evidence to address those questions (Chapter 3); and appraising the evidence, whether from qualitative, quantitative, or mixed-methods research, or a systematic review or clinical guidelines (Chapters 4 to 8), but also your skills in using clinical judgment to apply evidence in making clinical decisions with individual patients (Chapter 9). This requires careful consideration of the patient's individual needs, circumstances, and preferences and a recognition that how we communicate to patients affects their decisions (all crucial components of EBP), as well as an understanding of the potential for the research findings to be generalizable to that patient in that context. In the final chapter, we consider EBP in the context of organizational culture (Chapter 10). Here we examine the national and local initiatives that instill an organizational culture that promotes decisions that appropriately weigh research evidence, patient preference, available resources, and clinical expertise at all levels of healthcare systems. All chapters offer you the opportunity to consolidate your learning by completing online exercises, for which example solutions are provided. The exercise for Chapter 1 can be accessed via http://evolve.elsevier.com/Craig/evidence/.

References

American Association of Colleges of Nursing (AACN), 2006. The essentials of doctoral education for advanced nursing practice. Available from: http://www.aacnnursing.org/Portals/42/Publications/DNPEssentials.pdf (Accessed 01.05.18.).

American Association of Colleges of Nursing (AACN), 2008. The essentials of baccalaureate education for professional nursing practice. Available from: http://www.aacnnursing.org/ Portals/42/Publications/BaccEssentials08.pdf (Accessed 01.05.18.).

American Association of Colleges of Nursing (AACN), 2011. The essentials of master's education in nursing. Available from: https://www.aacnnursing.org/Portals/42/Publications/MastersEssentials11.pdf (Accessed 01.05.18.).

Campbell, J.M., Umapathysivam, K., Xue, Y., Lockwood, C., 2015. Evidence-based practice point-of-care resources: a quantitative evaluation of quality, rigor, and content. Worldviews Evid. Based Nurs. 12 (6), 313–327.

Canadian Nurses Association, 2017. Code of ethics for registered nurses. ISBN: 978-1-55119-441-7. Available from: https://www.cna-aiic.ca/-/media/cna/page-content/pdf-en/code-of-ethics-2017-edition-secure-interactive.pdf (Accessed 14.06.18.).

Castro-Sánchez, E., Holmes, A.H., 2015. Impact of organizations on healthcare-associated infections. J. Hosp. Infect. 89 (4), 346–350.

Correa-de-Araujo, R., 2016. Evidence-based practice in the United States: challenges, progress, and future directions. Health Care Women Int. 37 (1), 2–22.

Cronenwett, L., Sherwood, G., Barnsteiner, J., Disch, J., Johnson, J., Mitchell, P., et al., 2007. Quality and safety education for nurses. Nurs. Outlook 55 (3), 122–131.

Department of Health, 2001. Working Together – Learning Together: A Framework for Lifelong Learning for the NHS. Department of Health, London.

Department of Health, 2003. Winning Ways. Working Together to Reduce Healthcare Associated Infection in England. Department of Health, London.

Department of Health, 2008. High Quality Care for All: NHS Next Stage Review Final Report. Department of Health, London.

Department of Health, 2009. High Quality Care for All: Our Journey So Far. Department of Health, London.

Eccles, M.P., Mittman, B.S., 2006. Welcome to implementation science. Implement Sci 1, 1. Available from: https://doi.org/10.1186/1748-5908-1-1>.

Echevarria, I.M., Teegarden, G., Kling, J., 2017. Promoting a culture of evidence-based practice through a change request process. Nurse Lead 15 (4), 281–285.

Eriksson, T., Lu, H., Wiffen, P., 2014. Chapter 6: how to best practice evidence-based pharmacy with your available resources? Eur. J. Hosp. Pharm. 21, 194–201.

European Centre for Disease Prevention and Control, 2013, 2013. Point prevalence survey of healthcare-associated infections and antimicrobial use in European acute care hospitals. ECDC, Stockholm. Available from: <https://www.ecdc.europa.eu/sites/portal/files/media/en/publications/Publications/healthcare-associated-infections-antimicrobial-use-PPS.pdf> (Accessed 28.10.18.).

Grahame Smith, D., 1998. Evidence based medicine: challenging the authority. J. R. Soc. Med. 35 (Suppl.), 7–11.

Greenhalgh, T., Howick, J., Maskrey, N., 2014. Evidence based medicine: a movement in crisis? BMJ 348, g3725. https://doi.org/10.1136/bmj.g3725.

Hessels, A.J., Larson, E.L., 2016. Relationship between patient safety climate and standard precaution adherence: a systematic review of the literature. J. Hosp. Infect. 92 (4), 349–362.

Institute of Medicine, 2000. To Err Is Human: Building a Safer Health System. National Academies Press, Washington, DC.

Institute of Medicine, 2001. Crossing the Quality Chasm: A New Health System for the 21st Century. National Academies Press, Washington, DC.

Institute of Medicine, 2003. Health Professions Education: A Bridge to Quality. National Academies Press, Washington, DC.

Institute of Medicine, 2008. Knowing What Works in Healthcare: A Roadmap for the Nation. National Academies Press, Washington, DC.

Institute of Medicine (US), 2011. Committee on Standards for Developing Trustworthy Clinical Practice Guidelines. In: Graham, R., Mancher, M., Miller Wolman, D., et al. (Eds.), National Academies Press (US); Chapter 4, Current Best Practices and Proposed Standards for Development of Trustworthy Clinical Practice Guidelines: Part 1, Getting Started. Clinical Practice Guidelines We Can Trust, Washington (DC). Available from: https://www.ncbi.nlm.nih.gov/books/NBK209537/ (Accessed 28.10.18.).

Iowa Model Collaborative, Buckwalter, K.C., Cullen, L., Hanrahan, K., Kleiber, C., McCarthy, A.M., Rakel, B., Authored on behalf of the Iowa Model Collaborative, et al., 2017. Iowa Model of Evidence-Based Practice: revisions and validation. Worldviews Evid. Based Nurs. 14 (3), 175–182.

Kalogianni, A., 2011. Factors affect in patient adherence to medication regimen. Health Sci. J. 5 (3), 157–158.

Madhavji, A., Araujo, E.A., Beom Kim, K., Buschang, P.H., 2011. Attitudes, awareness, and barriers toward evidence-based practice in orthodontics. Am. J. Orthod. Dentofacial Orthop. 140 (3), 309.e2316.e2.

Magill, S.S., Edwards, J.R., Bamberg, W., Beldavs, Z.G., Dumyati, G., Kainer, M.A., et al., 2014. Multistate point-prevalence survey of health care–associated infections. N. Engl. J. Med. 370 (13), 1198–1208.

Mathes, T., Jaschinski, T., Pieper, D., 2014. Adherence influencing factors - a systematic review of systematic reviews. Arch. Public Health 72 (1), 37.

Mauger, B., Marbella, A., Pines, E., Chopra, R., Black, E.R., Aronson, N., 2014. Implementing quality improvement strategies to reduce healthcare-associated infections: a systematic review. Am. J. Infect. Control 42 (Suppl. 10), S274–S283.

Melnyk, B.M., Fineout-Overholt, E., Stillwell, S.B., Williamson, K.M., 2010. Evidence-based practice: step by step. The seven steps of evidence-based practice: following this progressive, sequential approach will lead to improved health care and patient outcomes. Am. J. Nurs. 110 (1), 51–53.

Melnyk, B.M., Gallagher-Ford, L., Long, L.E., Fineout-Overholt, E., 2014. The establishment of evidence-based practice competencies for practicing registered nurses and advanced practice nurses in real-world clinical settings: proficiencies to improve healthcare quality, reliability, patient outcomes, and costs. World-views Evid. Based Nurs. 11 (1), 5–15.

Moja, L., Kwag, K.H., Lytras, T., Bertizzolo, L., Brandt, L., Pecoraro, V., et al., 2014. Effectiveness of computerized decision support systems linked to electronic health records: a systematic review and meta-analysis. Am. J. Public Health 104 (12), e12–e22.

Muir Gray, J.A., 1997. Evidence-Based Health Care: How to Make Health Policy and Management Decisions. Churchill Livingstone, New York.

Mulrow, C.D., 1995. Rationale for systematic reviews. In: Chalmers, I., Altman, D.G. (Eds.), Systematic Reviews. BMJ Publishing Group, London.

National Institute for Health and Clinical Excellence, 2012. Chapter 4: Developing review questions and planning the systematic review. In: The guidelines manual. National Institute for Health and Clinical Excellence, London. Available from: www.nice.org.uk (Accessed 28.10.18.).

NHS Health Research Authority Research Ethics Service, October 2017. Defining research. Available from: http://www.hra-decisiontools.org.uk/research/ (Accessed 05.11.18.).

Nilsen, P., 2015. Making sense of implementation theories, models and frameworks. Implement. Sci 10, 53. https://doi.org/10.1186/s13012-015-0242-0.

Nursing and Midwifery Board of Australia, 2016. 2016 Registered Nurse Standards for Practice. Available from: http://www.nursingmidwiferyboard.gov.au/Codes-Guidelines-Statements/Professional-standards/registered-nurse-standards-for-practice.aspx (Accessed 14.06.18.).

Nursing and Midwifery Council, 2018. The Code. Professional standards of practice and behavior for nurses and midwives. NMC, London. Available from: www.nursingcouncil.org.nz (Accessed 28.10.18.).

Nursing Council of New Zealand, 2012. 2012 Code of Conduct for Nurses. ISBN: 978-0-908662-45-6. Available from: www.nursingcouncil.org.nz. (Accessed 14.06.18.).

Pearson, M., 2000. Making a difference through research: how nurses can turn the vision into reality (editorial). NT Research 5 (2), 85–86.

QSEN Quality and Safety Education for Nurses, 2010. About QSEN. Available from: http://qsen.org/about-qsen/ (Accessed 2.10.10.).

Rotter, M.L., 1997. 150 years of hand disinfection. Semmelweis' heritage, 22. Hygiene und Medizin, pp. 332–339.

Sackett, D., Richardson, W.S., Rosenberg, W., Haynes, R.B., 1997. Evidence Based Medicine: How to Practice and Teach EBM. Churchill Livingstone, New York.

Sackett, D., Straus, S.E., Richardson, W.S., Rosenberg, W., Haynes, R.B., 2000. Evidence-Based Medicine. How to Practise and Teach EBM, second ed. Churchill Livingstone, London.

Schaffer, M.A., Sandau, K.E., Diedrick, L.J., 2013. Evidence-based practice models for organizational change: overview and practical applications. Adv. Nurs. 69 (5), 1197–1209.

Scurlock-Evans, L., Upton, P., Upton, D., 2014. Evidence-based practice in physiotherapy: a systematic review of barriers, enablers and interventions. Physiotherapy 100 (3), 208–219.

Shenoy, P., Harugeri, A., 2015. Elderly patients' participation in clinical trials. Perspect. Clin. Res. 6 (4), 184–189.

Stevens, K.R., 2004. ACE Star Model of EBP: knowledge transformation. Academic Center for Evidence-based Practice The University of Texas Health Science Center, San Antonio. Available from: www.acestar.uthscsa.edu (Accessed 28.10.18.).

Stevens, K.R., Staley, J., 2006. The quality chasm reports, evidence-based practice, and nursing's response to improve healthcare. Nurs. Outlook 54 (2), 94–101.

Stevens, K.R., 2009. Essential competencies for evidence-based practice in nursing, second ed. Academic Center for Evidence-based Practice (ACE) of University of Texas Health Science Center, San Antonio.

Stevens, K.R., McDuffie, K., Clutter, P.C., 2009. Research and the mandate for evidence-based practice, quality, and safety. In: Mateo, M., Kirchhoff, K. (Eds.), Research for Advance Practice Nurses: From Evidence to Practice. Springer Publishing Company, New York, pp. 43–70.

Titler, M., Kleiber, C., Steelman, V., Rakel, B.A., Budreau, G., Everett, L.Q., et al., 2001. The Iowa model of evidence-based practice to promote quality care. Crit. Care Nurs. Clins. North Am. 13 (4), 497–509.

Upton, D., Stephens, D., Williams, B., Scurlock-Evans, L., 2014. Occupational therapists' attitudes, knowledge, and implementation of evidence-based practice: a systematic review of published research. Br. J. Occup. Ther. 77 (1), 24–38.

Vangeli, E., Bakhshi, S., Baker, A., Fisher, A., Bucknor, D., Mrowietz, U., Östör, A.J., et al., 2015. A systematic review of factors associated with non-adherence to treatment for immune-mediated inflammatory diseases. Adv. Ther. 32 (11), 983–1028.

Veeramah, V., 2016. The use of evidenced-based information by nurses and midwives to inform practice. J. Clin. Nurs. 253 (3-4), 340–350.

Zimlichman, E., Henderson, D., Tamir, O., Franz, C., Song, P., Yamin, C.K., et al., 2013. Health care–associated infections: a meta-analysis of costs and financial impact on the US health care system. JAMA Intern. Med. 173 (22), 2039–2046.

How to Ask the Right Question

Jean V. Craig

Introduction

The process for ensuring that clinical decisions are, as far as possible, informed by current research evidence is not new. As described by Sackett et al. (2000), it entails:

1. Converting information needs about clinical problems into clear questions
2. Seeking evidence to answer those questions
3. Evaluating (critically appraising) the evidence for its validity (truthfulness) and usefulness
4. Integrating findings with clinical expertise, patient needs, and patient preferences to reach a decision as to the optimum course of action, and then applying this decision
5. Evaluating performance (and the outcome of the decision)

This approach is driven by the belief that up-to-date, well-conducted research, when used judiciously to inform clinical decisions, can help to improve patient outcomes.

An important first step of the process is to be clear about what information is needed to inform an aspect of nursing care, and to translate that information need into an explicit and succinct question that will drive the subsequent steps of the process. A carefully formulated question maximizes the likelihood that relevant evidence, where available, is identified and incorporated appropriately into the decision-making process. Where questions are poorly defined or where a haphazard approach is used to find papers, the likely result is non-focused reading of literature that may or may not be relevant or applicable to the topic of interest. Developing clearly defined clinical questions is thus an invaluable skill for nurses aiming to integrate best research evidence with the other key elements of decision-making (clinical expertise, patient preferences and values, and resource availability) when caring for patients.

This chapter describes how to frame questions for interrogating the research evidence. It focuses on a commonly used format for question formulation and uses clinical examples to illustrate its use.

Information for Effective Nursing Care

Nurses make numerous decisions when caring for their patients. Consider the following examples of nursing care/interventions carried out during the course of a morning by a nurse working in a general practice:

- Holding an asthma clinic for teenagers, some of whom have frequent acute exacerbations of asthma
- Performing a Pap/cervical smear test
- Advising a young man on interventions to alleviate acute lower back pain
- Discussing lifestyle choices with a patient who has type 2 diabetes mellitus

The information that the nurse needs for managing each of these clinical episodes is extensive and varied. To successfully advise teenagers on asthma management, the nurse needs an understanding of the pathology of asthma (think of this as foundational or background information needs); the environmental substances or particles that may irritate the airways; the effectiveness and comparative benefits and harms of each of the available interventions; and how well they are tolerated or accepted by patients (think of these as more specific, foreground information needs). Foundational (background) information, although not static, does not always change rapidly, so when nurses need to refresh their memories, textbooks might be a suitable resource for accessing such information. In contrast, foreground information is best obtained from recent publications of evidence-based guidelines, systematic reviews, or, in their absence, individual research studies. Ideally, this evidence will have been evaluated for local relevance and practicality by, for example, the organizational policy and procedural committee and, where appropriate, incorporated into the standards, protocols, or guidelines within the organization. It can then be routinely used to help inform clinical decisions. However, this is not the case with all questions.

The starting point for successfully tracking down foreground research evidence is the focused "answerable" question. Some of the questions that our practice nurse might have when caring for his or her patients are presented in Box 2.1.

BOX 2.1 ■ Examples of Information Needed

- Why do some patients with asthma have frequent attacks?
- What reasons do people give for avoiding taking preventative asthma medication?
- How can I help a patient to reach an informed decision on managing their asthma medications?
- What is the best method of administering the asthma drugs?
- Do cervical smear tests with normal results accurately exclude cervical cancer?
- What advice should I give to this person with back pain?
- What is the best way of monitoring for complications of diabetes?
- What is the most effective way of helping patients with diabetes to increase their level of physical activity?

Let's consider the nurses' questions relating to asthma. Teenagers may differ from older adults in their reasons for not taking preventative asthma medication, and the approach to helping these two groups decide how best to manage their asthma medication may therefore also need to differ. The most useful evidence to help inform medication management in teenagers is likely to come from research undertaken in teenagers, although research undertaken in other age groups may also be useful. The asthma-related questions listed in Box 2.1 do not specify an age group, and there is a chance that the more precise evidence from a teenage population may be overlooked, or not given enough consideration when deciding on clinical practice. Using a framework to build a focused question can help to ensure that the precise items of information that are needed to solve a problem are included in the question, and thus in the subsequent steps of an evidence-based approach to health care, as discussed in the following sections.

Turning Information Needs into Focused Questions

As with the process of *doing* research, the process of *using* research flows from the question. When conducting research, the study design and methods are determined by what the researcher wants to know, that is, by the research question. Similarly, when aiming to use best available evidence in clinical decision-making, it is the clinical question that drives each step of the process; it guides the search for relevant evidence, it guides which study designs are likely to provide the most valid evidence, and helps to frame whether the identified evidence is applicable to the patients and setting in which it is to be used. We will look at each of these in more detail.

Searching for Evidence

The key components of the clinical question inform the strategy for searching for research evidence. When searching electronic databases that contain healthcare publications, such as CINAHL, MEDLINE, Embase, and the Cochrane Library databases, the more explicit the question, the easier it is to design an effective and efficient search strategy, that is, a search that readily yields the required information. This is discussed in detail in Chapter 3.

Selecting Evidence Based on Study Design

Once the question has been formulated, the type of study design that will best answer that question becomes clear. Chapters 4,5 and 6 discuss different types of qualitative, quantitative and mixed methods study designs, respectively, and Chapter 7 discusses systematic reviews. For the moment, it is sufficient to know that certain study designs are considered to be more appropriate for certain types of question, and studies identified by the search can be sifted accordingly:

- A question about the effectiveness of a treatment is best addressed by a well-conducted systematic review of randomized controlled trials (RCTs), or by a RCT in which participants are randomly allocated to receive or not receive an intervention, with the groups being followed up for the outcome event of interest. The point of randomization is that it reduces the risk of allocation bias (which could occur if the researchers influence which treatment group the participants are allocated to) and, thereby, confounding (differences between treatment groups in baseline characteristics that influence treatment and outcome measures) (Sedgwick, 2012).
- Where information about the prognosis of a disease (i.e., possible outcomes of a disease and the frequency of these outcomes) is required, the best evidence would be provided by a good-quality cohort study (Thiese, 2014). Patient characteristics (e.g., age or weight) or things to which patients are exposed (e.g., processed foods, secondhand smoke) that are strongly associated with a particular outcome are called *prognostic factors*. It may be

---

BOX 2.2 ■ Examples of Optimal Study Designs According to Clinical Question

Questions about effectiveness of an intervention
   Randomized controlled trial (or systematic review thereof)
Questions about the accuracy of a diagnostic test
   Studies that compare the new test against a reference standard test
Questions about prognosis
   Cohort studies or, when the outcome is rare or the required duration of follow-up is long, case-control studies
Questions about etiology (causation)
   Case-control or cohort study
Questions about perceptions, attitudes, beliefs, and experiences
   Qualitative research (numerous approaches)

---

impossible or unethical to randomize patients to different prognostic factors, and so the RCT is not an appropriate study design for investigating prognosis. Instead, a cohort study is conducted in which groups (cohorts) with and without the exposure or prognostic factor of interest are followed forward in time to see how many people in each group develop the specified outcome (e.g., cancer).

■ Case-control studies are useful for establishing prognosis in rare conditions or when a long follow-up is required (Thiese, 2014), and to investigate etiology (cause) of a disease. Participants who have already developed the specified outcome event (cases) are compared with participants who do not have the same outcomes (controls). Researchers look back in time to assess their history and to establish the percentage of "cases" and "controls" that have experienced the exposure of interest. For a graphical representation of the difference between cohort and case-control studies you may wish to look at the paper by Song and Chung (2010).

■ For a question relating to a patient's understanding of his or her condition or experiences of undergoing an intervention, we would look for well-conducted qualitative studies, of which there are numerous approaches. Regardless of the approach, qualitative research is committed to viewing the phenomenon of interest from the perspective of the people being studied (Ravitch and Mittenfelner, 2016), and thus aims to give insight into the different meanings and values that people may attribute to "events."

Box 2.2 provides a flavor of different types of questions and preferred study designs.

It is important to note at this point that the ideal source of evidence to guide clinical decisions comprises up-to-date clinical guidelines, which may be in the form of "bundles" (small sets of evidence-based processes or elements that, when performed together, improve patient outcome) (Resar et al., 2005) that have been informed by pre-synthesized, current, high-quality evidence of the most appropriate design, and adopted into organizational practice. If you identify a guideline that addresses your information needs, you can check whether the types of study designs underpinning each recommendation are appropriate. This will help you to judge how much confidence you can place in the recommendations. Guidelines and bundles have often been developed by notable organizations such as the American Heart Association, the Institute for Healthcare Improvement, and the National Institute for Health and Care Excellence. Chapter 8 discusses guidelines in more detail.

Understanding the Applicability of the Evidence

A judgment has to be made as to whether the results from the research would be achieved if they were applied to the specific patient group in your setting. It is unlikely that the circumstances in which the research study was undertaken will exactly match your clinical situation, and this may

---

BOX 2.3 ■ The Five-Part Question (PICOS)

Patient, population, or problem

Define who or what the question is about. *Tip: describe a group of patients similar to yours.*

Intervention or exposure

Define which intervention or exposure you are interested in. An intervention is a planned course of action (e.g., an educational package, a wound dressing, a smoking-cessation intervention). An exposure is something that happens (e.g., a fall, anxiety, exposure to house dust mites). *Tip: describe what it is you are considering doing or what the patient group has experienced or been exposed to.*

Comparison intervention (if any)

Define the alternative intervention. *Tip: this may be current practice or an alternative type of intervention used as a comparator. You may not have a comparator, in which case leave this blank.*

Outcome

Define the important outcomes, beneficial and/or harmful. *Tip: Define what you are hoping to achieve or avoid.*

Study design

Define the types of study design that would best answer the question. *Tip: there may be more than one appropriate study design, for example if the outcomes of interest are both "effectiveness" and "patient experience," then RCTs (and systematic reviews of RCTs) and qualitative research study designs would be of interest.*

---

affect the applicability or transferability of the study results. When reading a research study, it is important to decide whether the setting and participants included in the study are so dissimilar from your setting and patient group that the results cannot be applied. Is it appropriate, for example, to apply the findings of a study that looked at methods for improving adherence to drug treatment in the elderly to a population of teenagers? Methods that are effective in the elderly, such as the dispensing of tablets into individual containers labeled with the days of the week, may be seen by adolescents as embarrassing and may in fact result in reduced compliance. Similarly, a judgment must be made as to whether a similar, but not identical, intervention or test is likely to produce the same result as that achieved in the study.

As shown later in this chapter, the carefully formulated question usually includes a description of the patient group of interest, the planned treatment(s) or investigation(s), and the key outcomes that the patient hopes to achieve. It is therefore a useful tool for screening out those research studies that are unlikely to be applicable to the clinical situation or patient group.

A Framework for Formulating Questions

The PICOS (population, intervention, comparison intervention, outcome, study design) question framework, devised by Sackett et al. (1997), remains a commonly used approach for building a focused clinical question (Box 2.3). The framework helps to fine-tune the clinical question through encouraging clarification of each item needed to address the particular information need. This should be done in advance of seeking out research evidence.

Variations on PICOS include PICO(T)S, where the T refers to the time frame for attaining or sustaining the outcome of interest, in other words, the time point at which the outcome of interest should ideally have been measured in a research study (Riva et al., 2012), and PICO(D)S, where D refers to the digital method of assessing the outcome (where relevant) (Sisson, 2017). These variations can be used as prompts to encourage a more thorough consideration of the outcomes. Careful thought is required when deciding how general or specific each part of the question should be.

In terms of **population,** your goal may be to find evidence from research conducted in patients with a specific disease regardless of their age, gender, disease severity, or co-morbidities. However, there may be good reasons for restricting your search to studies undertaken in a more "select" group of patients. This will depend on whether or not the results of studies undertaken in a broad, inclusive research population would be generalizable to your specific patient group. To illustrate, there may be good clinical reasons for suspecting that the results from studies conducted in newly diagnosed patients are unlikely to be applicable to patients with long-standing disease. By recognizing that your population of interest comprises those with long-standing disease, you can devise a search strategy that targets studies undertaken in this population (e.g., using the search term "chronic"). Also, when sorting through the studies retrieved by the search, you can immediately put to one side those publications that report on newly diagnosed patients only. Of course, such studies may provide some useful information, but if good-quality studies are available that investigate patients with long-standing conditions, why bother with them?

It is helpful to think through the exact nature of the **intervention** (or test or exposure) that you are interested in learning about and the **comparison intervention** (if any). This is especially important for multifaceted interventions such as asthma clinics or behavioral change interventions, where any number of factors may be responsible for the outcome of interest. Describing the duration or frequency of the intervention and the method of applying the intervention may be an important factor in helping you select studies that have investigated an intervention that best matches one that you are considering providing. However, you may want to be less prescriptive here, particularly if there is scope for you to adapt your intervention to match any research-proven interventions identified in the search.

Deciding on the most important **outcomes** is not always straightforward, but can be facilitated by considering the patient's perspective alongside the perspectives of the healthcare practitioner and funder. The point here is that you want to seek out studies that have investigated important outcomes—not just studies that have investigated easy-to-measure but non-informative outcomes—using appropriate methods of measurement, undertaken at sensible time points.

Knowing which type of **study design** would best answer the question enables a more restricted search (i.e., the search can be tailored to seek out studies of a specific design) and also enables rapid sorting of the retrieved studies such that studies with the most appropriate study design take precedence. Be aware that researchers are not always able to apply the preferred study design in their research due to prohibitive costs, time restrictions, or ethical considerations, and might have had to resort to less than optimal study designs. We have mentioned previously that the ideal scenario would be to identify a current evidence-based guideline that is explicitly informed by studies of the most appropriate design.

APPLYING THE PICOS QUESTION FRAMEWORK

PICOS is particularly useful for framing questions about the effectiveness of interventions as illustrated in the following scenarios.

SCENARIO 2.1

A 10-year-old girl who has had open-heart surgery has been very ill for 2 days, requiring artificial ventilation and a number of support drugs to maintain her blood pressure. She has developed a small pressure injury at the back of her head.

The nurse asks the following question:

What more should we do to prevent pressure injuries in children in intensive care?

Many factors contribute to tissue breakdown, including poor nutrition, poor circulation, immobility, and type of mattress. The nurse is specifically interested in types of mattresses. The intensive care unit currently uses high-specification foam mattresses in most patients, but also has access to a small number of pressure-redistribution mattresses.

The PICOS question framework helps with thinking through each "component" of the question.

Population

The nurse must decide whether research carried out in the adult population could be applied to children. The decision of whether to exclude specific age groups is usually based on the known or inferred differences in the response to disease, treatments, and tests, by each age group. If the differences are such that the results of a research study will not be generalizable from one age group to another, then age groups should be defined within the question. In this case, the nurse decides that although evidence from adults may be generalizable to children, a first step would be to seek out evidence from studies in children.

In addition, it is important to consider whether there is any reason for restricting the question to patients who have had cardiac surgery. Critically ill cardiac patients may have poor circulation and, therefore, be at increased risk of developing pressure injury; however, other groups of critically ill children, for example children with septicemia, might also have poor perfusion. One could argue that all critically ill children are at increased risk of developing pressure injuries, and research carried out in these patients, regardless of their diagnosis, would help to answer the question.

Intervention (or Test or Exposure)

A variety of mattresses and beds are available on the market, ranging from standard foam or high-specification foam, to constant low-pressure mattresses, to mattresses that mechanically alternate the amount of pressure applied. Some of these mattresses may be more effective than others. Depending on the mattress under consideration, there could be major cost implications (Shi et al., 2018), so careful consideration of their effectiveness is important. The nurse decides to search for studies that have investigated any type of pressure-alternating mattresses. A few such mattresses are already available on the unit.

Comparison

It is not always necessary to define a comparison intervention, but in this case the intervention against which the proposed device could be compared is the method currently in use, the high-specification foam mattress.

Outcome

The nurse is seeking evidence on how to reduce the risk of patients developing pressure injuries and should therefore look for studies that report the incidence of pressure injuries. Pressure injuries are localized injuries to the skin that may also extend to the underlying tissue, which usually appear over a bony prominence or where an object or device presses against the skin (Edsberg et al., 2016). They can progress in severity at a fairly rapid rate. Information on the incidence of early-stage pressure injuries would therefore be just as useful to the nurse as information on the incidence of more severe injuries. The nurse decides to include studies in which the outcome includes pressure injuries that appear to fit any of the definitions included in the International Pressure Injury Staging System (Edsberg et al., 2016).

In summary, the key components of the question are:
- *Population:* Critically ill children
- *Intervention:* Pressure-alternating mattresses
- *Comparison:* High-specification foam mattresses
- *Outcome:* Pressure injuries at any stage/severity

■ *Study design:* As this is a question about the effectiveness of a therapy, the study design most likely to provide a valid answer to the question is a systematic review of RCTs or an RCT, or, ideally, a guideline that is explicitly informed by evidence from these study designs. Retrieved studies can be sorted accordingly, with studies of the above design being given highest priority.

The question is: In critically ill children, are pressure-alternating mattresses more effective than high-specification foam mattresses in preventing pressure injuries (at any stage/severity)?

Searching for research evidence is covered in detail in Chapter 3, but it is worth briefly mentioning here that it is not always necessary or, indeed, desirable to use all four parts of the question when developing a search strategy. The nurse could run a preliminary search using terms from the *population* ("child," "critically ill") and *intervention* ("pressure-alternating mattresses") parts of the question. If this does not readily yield relevant references, terms from one of the other components could be added. A filter could be added to the search so that only studies of a particular design are retrieved. Search filters are discussed in Chapter 3.

The nurse will be able to check the retrieved articles against the focused question. Those that are found to be less applicable can be set aside in favor studies that are generalizable to the 10-year-old child.

We have looked at one question in detail, but other questions that might arise from this scenario are highlighted in Table 2.1. The final example in the table shows a broad question: the nurse is hoping to find any key articles about pressure injury prevention to update his or her general knowledge.

TABLE 2.1 ■ **Further Questions About Prevention or Treatment of Pressure Injuries**

Population or Problem	Intervention (or Test or Exposure)	Comparison Intervention (If Any)	Outcome	Study Design
Patients with pressure injuries (at any stage)	Application of hydrocolloid dressing	Application of gauze dressing	Time to healing Time to shrinkage of the pressure injury Cost	Systematic review of RCTs or an RCT or, ideally, a guideline*
Patients with pressure injuries (at any stage)	Usual diet plus ascorbic acid supplementation	Usual diet with no additional supplements	Time to healing Time to shrinkage of the pressure injury	As above
Critically ill children	Pressure-alternating mattress with two-hourly turning	Pressure-alternating mattress alone	Incidence of pressure injuries (any stage) Risk of destabilizing the patient, poor cardiac output Comfort and acceptability	As above Further information on comfort and acceptability could be sought from studies with a qualitative design
Adults and children in any setting	Interventions of any type to prevent pressure injury	Not defined	Incidence of pressure injuries (any stage) Costs Comfort and acceptability	As above

*The guideline should be explicitly informed by evidence from the stipulated study designs.

SCENARIO 2.2

Alison, a 2-year-old girl, presented at the local emergency department with fever and vomiting. The attending doctor wondered if she might have a urinary tract infection (UTI). In line with departmental policy, urine was collected in a bag (which had been applied to her perineum according to the manufacturer's instructions) and then sent for microscopy and culture. The white blood cell count was found to be high, and Alison was started on a course of antibiotics. She was asked to return in a few days, by which time the urine culture results would be available. At her follow-up appointment, the attending physician was frustrated to note that the culture results showed a mixed growth. It was not clear whether Alison had indeed suffered a UTI or whether the urine sample had simply been contaminated. Children with possible UTI are investigated carefully. Untreated UTIs can cause renal scarring, chronic kidney disease, and sepsis (although we note a recent paper has questioned this view; damage to kidney tissue has been found to be congenital in some cases) (Okarska-Napierała et al., 2017).

Concerned that the methods used for obtaining urine samples were inappropriate, the physician suggested that, in future, bag-catch urine sampling should be abandoned in favor of clean-catch urine sampling. This method requires that the infant's diaper is removed and the carer is provided with a sterile container and instructed to watch for the opportunity to catch the urine. The nurses on the unit were worried about the implications of changing practice. They felt that carers might not be successful in capturing urine specimens, and that this would cause delays for patients and their families.

The nurses want to know:

What is the best way of obtaining a urine specimen for culture, from a child?

We can check how focused the question is by examining each component individually.

Population

The population of interest comprises children suspected of having UTI; however, the nurses may want to consider further refining the population. The results of a study carried out on older children (who can more easily pass urine directly into a sterile collection pot) are likely to be different from those of a study carried out in children still wearing diapers.

Intervention (or Test or Exposure)

In this case, there are two interventions of interest: the method of urine sampling that is currently used (i.e., urine bag sampling) and the proposed method of "clean-catch" sampling. It may be useful to include brief details of the exact methods used when obtaining bag-catch and clean-catch urine specimens, as these may differ from those used by researchers, and this could affect the applicability of study results.

Comparison

Comparing two or more methods is a useful way of reaching a decision about a practice change. When investigating the accuracy of a (new) diagnostic test, the new test is compared against a reference standard test to see how well the two tests agree. A reference standard test is considered to be "the best available method for establishing the presence or absence of the condition of interest" and can be a single method or a combination of methods (Cohen et al., 2015; Naaktgeboren et al., 2013). Some reference standard tests are difficult to perform, invasive, costly, inconvenient, or unacceptable to the patient, which is why new tests are sought.

According to clinical guidelines of the American Academy of Pediatrics (updated in 2011), the reference standard method for obtaining urine from infants and babies with suspected UTI is urethral catheterization or suprapubic aspiration of urine directly from the bladder. These procedures are invasive, uncomfortable for the infant, and can be difficult to execute when infants are uncooperative.

TABLE 2.2 ■ Further Questions About Diagnosis of Urinary Tract Infection

Population or Problem	Intervention (or Test or Exposure)	Comparison Intervention (If Any)	Outcome	Study Design
Children suspected of having UTI, who are not yet toilet trained	Clean-catch urine sampling using a sterile container	Urethral catheterization or suprapubic aspiration directly from the bladder	Culture contamination	Systematic review of diagnostic test performance studies or a diagnostic test performance study or, ideally, a guideline*
Obtaining urine samples from children who are not yet toilet trained	Clean-catch method	Bag-catch method	Time taken to successfully obtain urine sample Cost Acceptability to patient, parent, nurse	Systematic review of RCTs or an RCT or, ideally, a guideline* Further information on acceptability could be sought from studies with a qualitative design

*The guideline should be explicitly informed by evidence from the stipulated study designs.

Outcome

The key outcome of interest is contamination of the culture specimen.

In summary:

- *Population:* Children suspected of having UTI, who are not yet toilet trained
- *Interventions:* Bag-catch urine specimens and clean-catch urine specimens
- *Comparison:* Urethral catheterization or suprapubic aspiration
- *Outcome:* Contaminated culture specimen, as indicated by bacterial growth in either the bag-catch or clean-catch specimens, not found in the suprapubic aspiration.

The revised question is:

In children suspected of having UTI, who are not yet toilet trained, what is the risk of culture contamination when urine is obtained by (i) bag-catch or (ii) clean-catch, as compared with urine obtained by urethral catheterization or suprapubic aspiration directly from the bladder?

The optimal *study design* for this question would be studies assessing diagnostic test performance or accuracy (discussed in Chapter 5). Examples of additional questions relating to this scenario are given in Table 2.2.

Other Frameworks for Formulating Questions

PECOS

Once you are used to using PICOS to focus your questions, you may find that you start to adapt it slightly. We have sneaked in a slight adaptation in Box 2.3; we included both interventions and exposures under the **I** component of PICOS. We could instead have used PECOS to help focus questions about **e**xposures, as shown in this example adapted from Wikoff et al. (2017), who were concerned about the emergence of caffeine-containing energy drinks, dietary supplements, and food items, and wanted to ascertain whether high caffeine intake can adversely affect certain groups such as pregnant women, children, and adolescents.

In healthy pregnant women (P), is caffeine intake above 300 mg/day (E), compared with lower intakes (C), associated with adverse pregnancy outcomes such as miscarriage, stillbirth, or preterm birth (O)?

When seeking out research evidence to answer a question about the effects of exposure to a substance, we could look for the following study designs (S): cohort studies that follow the progress of a cohort of participants over a period of time to see whether, in the light of their exposure history (estimated caffeine intake), they develop the outcome of interest (adverse pregnancy outcomes); case control studies that look back in time to gather information from cases (women with adverse pregnancy outcomes) and controls (women without problems during pregnancy) to compare their exposure history (estimated caffeine intake). Chapter 5 explains this in more detail.

In this second example, a young man is discharged from an overnight stay in hospital, having sustained a mild traumatic brain injury after a fall from his horse. He has symptoms of concussion. He wants to know how long these symptoms are likely to persist. The focused question could be:

For patients of any age (P) diagnosed with mild traumatic brain injury (E), what proportion will have physical, cognitive, and/or emotional symptoms after 3 months (O)?

SPICE

When searching for research evidence to help us understand people's perspectives, decisions, behaviors, or experiences (this type of evidence is usually obtained from qualitative research, discussed in Chapter 4), we could use the SPICE question framework (Booth 2006) if we find it more intuitive than PICOS.

SPICE comprises $\underline{S}$etting, $\underline{P}$erspective, $\underline{I}$nterest (Phenomenon of), $\underline{C}$omparison, $\underline{E}$valuation

Here, the population part of the question has been separated into two parts: $\underline{S}$etting (where) and $\underline{P}$erspective (for whom). People's experiences and perceptions are subjective. Setting will have a substantial bearing on their lived experiences, behaviors, and beliefs. It is therefore useful to know what setting you are interested in as well as which stakeholder group is the focus. $\underline{I}$ is used for the phenomenon of interest (or an intervention such as a substance misuse rehabilitation program). $\underline{C}$ is the comparator (if any), and $\underline{E}$ is for evaluation (e.g., their knowledge about substance misuse programs, their experiences of being excluded from school, and what impact they believe this has had on their behavior).

An example of a focused question:

What do we know about the experiences (E) of adolescents (P) from areas of high deprivation (S) of being excluded from school due to substance misuse (I) and their views on how this impacts on their behavior (E)?

It's not essential to bring the information together as a question. You could simply write out the information under each letter (S, P, I, C, E). The important thing is to have a clear idea of your precise information needs.

SPIDER

This question framework, also used to identify qualitative research, was developed specifically for people undertaking systematic reviews of qualitative research (Cooke et al., 2012), and so we will give only very brief details here.

SPIDER comprises $\underline{S}$ample, $\underline{P}$henomenon of $\underline{I}$nterest, $\underline{D}$esign, $\underline{E}$valuation, and $\underline{R}$esearch type.

"$\underline{S}$ample" was considered by the authors to be a more relevant term than "Population," because findings from qualitative research are not always intended to be generalizable beyond the population included in the study (Cooke et al., 2012). $\underline{D}$esign refers to the theoretical framework (e.g., ethnography, phenomenology) or the method of obtaining data (e.g., focus groups, interview) and influences the strength of the study findings. $\underline{R}$esearch type refers to the broad research approach (e.g., qualitative, mixed methods). $\underline{C}$omparison is not included in this framework; the authors point out that because of the exploratory nature of qualitative work and the smaller samples, comparison groups are not routinely used.

ECLIPSE

This framework may be useful in building focused questions about health management topics (Wildridge and Bell, 2002).

ECLIPSE comprises Expectation (the service improvement needed), Client group (at whom the service is aimed), Location (where the service is located), Impact (the outcomes), Professionals (who is providing or improving the service), ServicE (the service of interest).

Prioritizing Questions

Change is constant: new technologies are introduced on a regular basis (e.g., e-technology such as a smoking-cessation app may take the place of, or be used as an adjunct to, face-to-face therapy; new drugs are introduced); healthcare settings can change (e.g., the usual place for caring for patients requiring long-term ventilation may change from the hospital setting to the home); and new information emerges (e.g., research unveils new understandings about prognostic factors for sudden infant death syndrome or about literacy figures for the adult population). A questioning approach to health care is important if such "innovations" are to be identified in the first place and then taken into consideration when managing patients. An attitude of continuously questioning the status quo should be encouraged (Echevarria et al., 2017), asking questions such as "Which is best?", "Who should do this?", and "Where should patients like this be treated?" Blind acceptance of a technology that is skillfully marketed, or outright rejection of change to an existing practice, could potentially negatively on patient outcome, resources, and cost. One of the challenges for nurses and other healthcare professionals is to recognize the importance of asking questions about healthcare practices.

It may be necessary to prioritize the questions for which best evidence is to be sought. Factors to consider include:

- Genuine uncertainty or controversy as to which course of action should be taken
- Wide variations in practice (among staff, units, settings)
- Suggestions by patients
- Unexpected outcomes
- New therapies, technologies, or management approaches becoming available
- Practices based on tradition and ritualistic practices (are they effective, cost effective, necessary?)
- Questions that arise repeatedly, possibly from a number of sources
- Questions that have potentially important consequences (e.g., risk, cost, resource use, staffing, impact on patient's well-being)
- Questions where there is potential to affect change

For those aspects of care that are already entrenched in day-to-day practice, a questioning approach is important, but can be difficult to achieve. Where a method of care delivery (e.g., the "drugs round" in which drugs are dispensed to all ward patients at set times by a designated nurse) has become entrenched as routine practice, practitioners may accept it as the right or only method, and alternatives may not be considered. It may be helpful for the nurse to use a long-established approach of considering whether "the right person is doing the right thing, in the right way, in the right place, at the right time, with the right result" (Graham, 1996). By asking this question, any information gaps will be highlighted. Finally, reflection, a strategy used within nursing to encourage learning from practical experiences (Helyer 2015, Royal College of Nursing, 2018), can be used as another method for identifying information needs. By reflecting on "critical incidents," any gaps in knowledge of current research findings can be identified.

Questions and Research Evidence Aren't Enough

Our day-to-day clinical decisions are influenced (consciously or unconsciously) by a number of factors (Box 2.4). Although each of these factors is influential in its own right, when used in isolation, they may result in inappropriate decisions. The application of scientific evidence without considered judgment results in a "cookbook" approach to health care, with nurses following "recipes" for care regardless of the patient's specific needs. In contrast, over-reliance on personal experience when making decisions can be equally damaging. For example, if practice nurses continue to recommend bed rest to people with non-specific lower back pain because it appears to have worked in the past, they will be ignoring established evidence that bed rest is less effective than staying active in reducing pain and improving an individual's ability to perform everyday activities (Oliveira et al., 2018).

Up-to-date, valid evidence that is directly relevant to the situation at hand needs to be integrated together with the other influencing factors to maximize the likelihood of the expected outcome being achieved.

Exercises

We encourage you to consolidate your learning by undertaking the exercises on the website, including the PICO-PICO game.

Summary

The success or failure of explicitly basing nursing practice on best evidence relies on nurses challenging both new and established methods of caring for patients. The skills provided in this

---

BOX 2.4 ■ Factors Influencing the Decision-Making Process

Up-to-date research evidence
Clinical expertise:
- Formal education
- Accumulated knowledge (journal articles, textbooks, press reports, expert opinion, advice from colleagues, clinical audit)
- Past experience built on a case-by-case basis
- Pattern recognition, intuition
- Most recent experience
- Skill level

Beliefs, attitudes, values, tradition
Routine, "the way things are done around here"
Factors relating to the patient and family:
- Clinical circumstances, co-morbid conditions
- Preferences, values, beliefs, attitudes, expectations, concerns
- Needs

Organizational factors
- National and local policies
- Service/resource availability
- Funding
- Equipment
- Time

BOX 2.5 ■ Quick Reference: Applying Your New Skills in Clinical Practice

- Consider what additional information is required when making a healthcare decision.
- Prioritize which information you need to address.
- Formulate a question.
- Focus the question using a framework such as PICOS.
  - Decide how specific or how general each part of the question needs to be.
  - Decide which study design is most likely to provide valid results.
- Refer to the focused question at each stage of the evidence-based process, for example, when searching for or appraising evidence and when considering whether the evidence is applicable to your situation.

---

chapter, summarized in Box 2.5, provide a starting point for seeking out good-quality evidence to support current practice or a change in practice. Numerous opportunities for practicing these skills will present themselves during the course of the workday. This first step in the evidence-based process is an important one, and nurses who take the time to develop carefully worded questions will be well rewarded at each stage in the process.

References

American Academy of Pediatrics, 2011. Urinary tract infection: clinical practice guideline for the diagnosis and management of the initial UTI in febrile infants and children 2 to 24 months. Pediatrics 128 (3), 595–610.

Booth, A., 2006. Clear and present questions: formulating questions for evidence based practice. Library Hi Tech. 24 (3), 355–368.

Cohen, J.F., Korevaar, D.A., Altman, D.G., Bruns, D.E., Gatsonis, C.A., Hooft, L., et al., 2016. 2015 STARD 2015 guidelines for reporting diagnostic accuracy studies: explanation and elaboration. BMJ Open 6 (11), e012799.

Cooke, A., Smith, D., Booth, A., 2012. Beyond PICO: the SPIDER tool for qualitative evidence synthesis. Qual. Health Res. 22 (10), 1435–1443.

Echevarria, I.M., Teegarden, G., King, J., 2017. Promoting a culture of evidence-based practice through a change request process. Nurse Lead. 15 (4), 281–285.

Edsberg, L.E., Black, J.M., Goldberg, M., McNichol, L., Moore, L., Sieggreen, M., 2016. Revised National Pressure Ulcer Advisory Panel Pressure Injury Staging System: Revised Pressure Injury Staging System. J. Wound Ostomy Continence Nurs. 43 (6), 585–597.

Graham, G., 1996. Clinically effective medicine in a rational health service. Health Director (June), pp. 11–12.

Helyer, R., 2015. Learning through reflection: the critical role of reflection in work-based learning. Journal of Work–Applied Management 7 (1), 15–27.

Naaktgeboren, C.A., Bertens, L.C., van Smeden, M., de Groot, J.A., Moons, K.G., Reitsma, J.B., 2013. Value of composite reference standards in diagnostic research. BMJ 347, f5605.

Oliveira, C.B., Maher, C.G., Pinto, R.Z., Traeger, A.C., Lin, C.C., Chenot, J.F., van Tulder, M., Koes, B.W., 2018. Clinical practice guidelines for the management of non-specific low back pain in primary care: an updated overview. Eur. Spine J. 27 (11), 2791–2803.

Okarska-Napierała, M., Wasilewska, A., Kuchar, E., 2017. Urinary tract infection in children: diagnosis, treatment, imaging–comparison of current guidelines. J. Pediatr. Urol. 13 (6), 567–573.

Ravitch, S.M., Mittenfelner, C.N., 2016. Qualitative Research: Bridging the Conceptual, Theoretical, and Methodological. Sage Publications, Los Angeles.

Resar, R., Pronovost, P., Haraden, C., Simmonds, T., Rainey, T., Nolan, T., et al., 2005. Using a bundle approach to improve ventilator care processes and reduce ventilator-associated pneumonia. Jt. Comm. J. Qual. Patient Saf. 31 (5), 243–248.

Riva, J.J., Malik, K.M., Burnie, S.J., Endicott, A.R., Busse, J.W., 2012. What is your research question? An introduction to the PICOT format for clinicians. J. Can. Chiropr. Assoc. 56 (3), 167–171.

Royal College of Nursing, 2018. Revalidation requirements: reflection and reflective discussion. Available at: https://www.rcn.org.uk/professional-development/revalidation/reflection-and-reflective-discussion.

Sackett, D.L., Richardson, W.S., Rosenberg, W., Haynes, R.B., 1997. Evidence-Based Medicine: How to Practice and Teach EBM. Churchill Livingstone, New York.

Sackett, D.L., Strauss, S.E., Richardson, W.S., Rosenberg, W., Haynes, R.B., 2000. Evidence-Based Medicine: How to Practice and Teach EBM, second ed. Churchill Livingstone, London.

Sedgwick, P., 2012. Why randomise in clinical trials? BMJ 345, e5584.

Shi, C., Dumville, J.C., Cullum, N., 2018. Support surfaces for pressure ulcer prevention: a network meta-analysis. PloS One 13 (2), e0192707.

Sisson, H., 2017. How helpful are mnemonics in the development of a research question? Nurse Res. 25 (3), 42–45.

Song, J.W., Chung, K.C., 2010. Observational studies: cohort and case-control studies. Plast. Reconstr. Surg. 126 (6), 2234–2242.

Thiese, M.S., 2014. Observational and interventional study design types; an overview. Biochem. Med. 24 (2), 199–210.

Wikoff, D., Welsh, B.T., Henderson, R., Brorby, G.P., Britt, J., Myers, E., et al., 2017. Systematic review of the potential adverse effects of caffeine consumption in healthy adults, pregnant women, adolescents, and children. Food Chem. Toxicol. 109 (1), 585–648.

Wildridge, V., Bell, L., 2002. How CLIP became ECLIPSE: a mnemonic to assist in searching for health policy/management information. Health Info. Libr. J. 19 (2), 113–115.

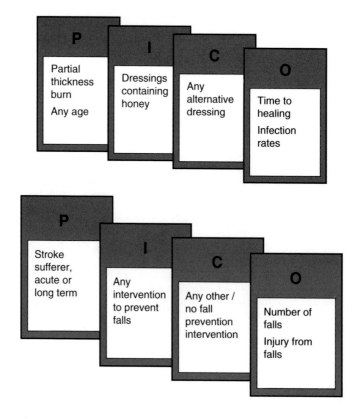

CHAPTER 3

Searching the Literature

Olwen Beaven ▪ Jean V. Craig

KEY POINTS

- Identifying best evidence requires an understanding of basic search principles. More advanced techniques will help to enhance a search.
- To identify research evidence in the most efficient way, start with a focused question, select databases that are most likely to yield the most useful information about your question, and build a search strategy using appropriate search terms, combined in the right way.
- Databases/resources are best searched in order of usefulness. If you can find pre-synthesized, pre-appraised evidence, this will save you a lot of work.
- Techniques to limit the number of irrelevant articles retrieved (such as searching using index terms only, where available) are invaluable.
- Systematic reviews require extensive searching, and it is advisable to obtain specialist advice on building comprehensive search strategies for each of the resources to be searched.

Introduction

This chapter provides a beginner's guide to the principles and practice of searching the research literature. Although it is unrealistic to teach the art of searching within the constraints of the printed page, it is possible to pass on a basic understanding of the search process and the core competencies needed for efficiently identifying research evidence to inform clinical decisions.

Although this chapter is primarily aimed at novice searchers, it provides useful revision for the more confident searcher and includes sections specifically for the advanced searcher.

We start the chapter with an overview of basic search principles applied to database searching and then discuss a systematic approach for retrieving the most useful evidence, targeting, for example, guidelines and "pre-appraised" synthesized evidence in the first instance. We present useful sources of evidence and show an example search on one of these sources (the MEDLINE PubMed database). We then give additional tips and techniques for refining a search and highlight the complexities of undertaking the comprehensive searching required for systematic review purposes.

Where Is Research Information Found?

The large number of journals produced around the world precludes searching for individual articles by hand. Journal indexes have therefore been converted onto electronic, bibliographic databases that gather together articles within a subject category such as engineering, sociology, history, medicine, or agriculture.

Databases are produced in a variety of formats; online or Internet versions and, in many organizations, databases are networked onto computers. Organizations have to pay to access databases, so a limited range may be made available in any one institution.

Most databases provide similar information about each included article (or "record"); usually the title, author, where it was published (the journal, year, volume, issue, page numbers), and the short abstract, if available. Databases do not normally contain the full text of the whole article although, increasingly, free full-text articles are becoming available electronically.

Each section of a journal article (e.g., title, author, abstract) in a database is called a "field." Each new field starts with a two-letter code to make it clearly identifiable. For example, a typical record in a bibliographic database might look something like this:

TI: The Joys of Nursing
AU: Anybody G.C., Somebody H.L., Other A.N.
SO: Supernurse, 2019, 15 (2); 378–84
PY: 2019
AB: There have been numerous campaigns to boost the recruitment of young people into the nursing profession. These have taken a variety of approaches and have focused on different aspects of the job, from the challenges experienced, to the rewards of supporting patients to recovery. This paper examines the positive images of nursing portrayed in these advertising campaigns and compares them with the reality as perceived by nurses currently employed.
UI: SN9725938

Getting Help with Database Searching

Hospital or university libraries are an obvious port of call for obtaining training, advice or self-help tutorials on literature searching. Librarians can help you focus your question, construct the search, and select which databases to search. Increasingly, librarians are offering an information service whereby they conduct the search for articles relevant to a clinical question. Such services are useful, but acquiring the skills to conduct your own searches will prove invaluable in terms of day-to-day clinical decision-making.

Basic Search Principles

Although databases are produced by different companies and vary in terms of subject matter and layout, they all require the same general approach to searching. The key principle in searching is to match words that describe your question or topic of interest with journal articles containing the same or similar words, in the hope that these journal articles will address your information needs. This section looks at some basic theory that can be applied to searching most databases.

ANALYZING THE QUESTION

When starting a literature search, it is important to have a clear question in mind so that the information required can be identified in the most efficient way. The first step in developing a search strategy is to tease out the key components of the question using PICOS (Population, Intervention, any Comparison interventions, intended Outcomes and optimum Study design to address the question). An example is given in Box 3.1. If you are looking for information to help you understand people's decisions, behaviors, or experiences, you could frame the question using SPIDER (Sample, Phenomenon of Interest, Design, Evaluation, Research type), or SPICE (Setting, Perspective, Interest (Phenomenon of), Comparison, Evaluation), as discussed in Chapter 2. In this chapter, we use PICOS for illustrative purposes.

BOX 3.1 ■ Key Components of a Question

Question: In people with needle phobia, what are the effects of non-pharmacologic interventions on their fear or anxiety associated with needles and injections?

Population:	People with fear of needles
Intervention(s):	Behavioral therapy (any type)
Comparison:	One behavioral therapy intervention compared with another
Outcome:	Fear/anxiety
Study Design:	Randomized controlled trial

BOX 3.2 ■ Suggested Word Lists for the Question on Needle Phobia

Population:	Fear, phobia
	Needles, syringes, injection(s), hypodermic(s)
Interventions:	Behavio(u)r(al) therapy, relaxation, coping skills, cognitive therapy, hypnotherapy, hypnosis, psychotherapy, distraction, diversion (and so on)
Comparison:	(Same as interventions)
Outcomes:	Alleviation or reduction of fear/stress/anxiety, stress relief, calm, relaxed
Study Design:	Randomized controlled(-)trial, randomised controlled(-)trial, RCT

SEARCH TERMS

Having established the key components of a question, generate a word list for each component.

Free Text

In free text searching, you build word lists of the different terms that authors may use to describe a key component of the search, including plural and singular words, synonyms, abbreviations, variations in spellings (e.g., UK "colour" and US "color") and possible hyphenation. Be cautious when using abbreviations. A search for articles using the abbreviation "AIDS," for example, will identify articles looking at hearing aids, mobility aids, and so on, and articles on autoimmune deficiency syndrome. If too many irrelevant articles are retrieved from a search incorporating abbreviations, consider re-running the search without the abbreviated terms. The lists for each component may be fairly comprehensive, as shown in Box 3.2.

Type the list of words for one or more of the PICOS components into the search window, combining the words with the appropriate linking word (as explained later in this chapter). The database then matches this combination of words to records containing the same words anywhere within the abstract, title, or author fields, or, in some databases, anywhere within the record.

A search using free text usually has a high recall rate or high sensitivity (large numbers of records are retrieved by the search), but a low precision rate or low specificity (many of the retrieved records are irrelevant) (National Health Service Centre for Reviews and Dissemination, 2001). This is because in free text searching, any record containing the free text words is retrieved, even if the words are used to discuss a minor detail within the record. To increase precision of the search, albeit at the expense of sensitivity, a search using index terms only (see later) can be carried out.

Controlled Vocabulary (Index) Searching

Index terms are keywords that are added onto each journal article by the database producers to reflect the most important topics covered in that article. For example, articles within a specific database that contain the terms "breast cancer," "breast carcinoma," or "breast tumor" will all be assigned the unique index term "breast neoplasm" by the database producers. Regardless of the words the author uses to describe the topic in the article, it will always be labeled with the index term "breast neoplasm" within that specific database. When searching for articles on this topic, instead of having to think of all the different terms that authors might use, as is the case with free text searching, the appropriate index term can be used instead.

A further benefit is that articles that briefly mention a topic will not be retrieved when index terms only are used. This is because index terms are assigned only to those topics that form a large part of the record. A search using index terms, also known as *controlled vocabulary searching*, is therefore more precise (has a higher specificity) than a search using free text terms. A disadvantage of using index terms only is that any records that have not been appropriately indexed by the database producers may be missed by the search.

To find the index term, access the thesaurus provided in the database (e.g., in PubMed/MEDLINE, the database uses MeSH or Medical Sub Headings). Further information is given in Step 2 of the example search of the MEDLINE database (PubMed version).

Combined Free Text and Controlled Vocabulary (Index) Searching

Some databases automatically match free text search terms to appropriate index terms, thereby retrieving records through a combination of free text and controlled vocabulary searching. The help section of the database will clarify whether this is done.

LINKING WORD LISTS USING BOOLEAN LOGIC: AND, OR, NOT

Search terms are linked together to get the combination of components needed for a question using the terms "AND" and "OR."

AND combines words together, so that both words must appear within one article to be found by a search (Fig. 3.1). A search for "needles AND fear" will find only those articles that contain both the words "needles" and "fear."

OR enables selection of any one of a number of specified words/phrases in a list, so that if either one or another specified word/phrase appears in an article, it will be found in a search (Fig. 3.2). A search for "relaxation OR hypnotherapy OR hypnosis OR distraction" will find articles containing at least one of the words/phrases in the list.

NOT excludes specific words from a search so articles containing them will not be identified (Fig. 3.3). A search for "heart NOT lung" will retrieve articles containing the word heart that do not also contain the word lung. If an initial search for articles on heart surgery retrieves numerous unwanted articles on combined heart and lung surgery, NOT could be used to exclude these unwanted articles. However, be cautious; potentially relevant articles on heart surgery that happen to mention lung will also be excluded.

AND, OR, and NOT, in this context, are known as "Boolean logic operators."

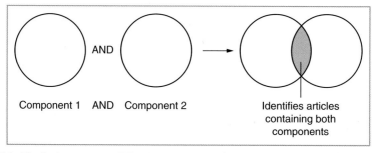

Fig. 3.1   The Boolean operator AND only identifies articles containing both specified components.

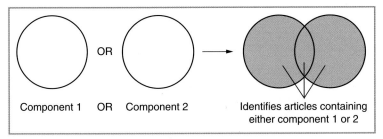

Fig. 3.2   The Boolean operator OR identifies articles containing either specified component.

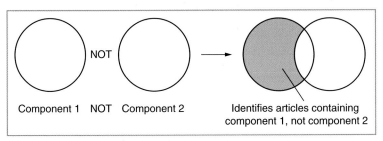

Fig. 3.3   The Boolean operator NOT identifies articles containing one specified component but not the other specified component.

ADDITIONAL SEARCH TECHNIQUES COMMONLY AVAILABLE
Phrase Searching

If you are looking for articles on, say, pressure ulcers, you will want to avoid retrieving articles that discuss pressure and ulcers separately, as such articles are unlikely to address your information need. In some databases, a search for the words pressure ulcer will retrieve records in which the words *pressure* and *ulcer* appear anywhere in the record, but not necessarily next to each other, thereby increasing the number of irrelevant records retrieved. For these databases, it is necessary to enclose the phrase in quotes ("pressure ulcer") or to use some other technique to force retrieval of articles that use the exact phrase "pressure ulcer." The Help option within the database will explain which technique to use.

Truncation

Many databases will retrieve only those records that contain the exact word that you have typed. Truncation avoids you having to type all the different variations of a word when free text searching. You type the stem of a word followed by the truncation symbol, often denoted by a * or $. The Help option within the database will explain which symbol should be used for truncation. A drawback is that truncation reduces the precision of the search:

- "ulcer$" would pick up ulcer, ulcers, ulceration, ulcerated, and so on (all potentially relevant to pressure ulcers), but also ulcer-carcinoma, ulcero-bubonic, and other words that have nothing to do with that topic.
- "Bab*" would pick up baby and babies, but also other words like baboon, babesiosis, Babinski, and so on.

Wildcard

The *wildcard*, available on some databases, allows you to search for words with alternative spellings without having to type each word in full. The wildcard is inserted in the word where extra or alternative letter(s) might be placed. It is often denoted by a "?" in databases:

- "an?emia" would pick up both anemia (US spelling) and anaemia (UK spelling).
- "wom?n" would pick up both woman and women.

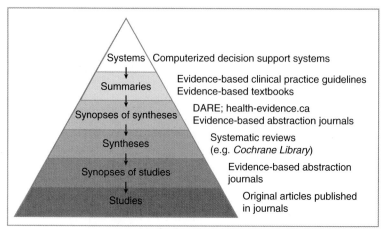

Fig. 3.4   The 6S model of pre-appraised evidence. (From DiCenso, A., Bayley, L., Haynes, B., 2009. Accessing pre-appraised evidence: fine-tuning the 5S model into a 6S model. Evid. Based Nurs. 12 [4], 99–101, with permission from BMJ Publishing Group.)

Where to Search

Having clarified a question and identified the words necessary to search for relevant information, the next step is to consider the resources most likely to contain articles relevant to that question.

It is tempting to dive online and see what can be found via an Internet browser. Although this simplicity is attractive, it is not the best way to identify well-conducted research evidence appropriate for use in clinical practice. The Internet is an unregulated resource. There is no quality control, so the information provided can be biased, unfounded, and misleading, just as easily as it can be accurate and well-balanced. Rather than exploring such a vast pool of information of unknown quality, it is preferable to take a structured approach that focuses on more reliable resources.

The 6S model, proposed by Haynes in 2001 and further refined by DiCenso et al. in 2009, remains a valid model for categorizing evidence-based information according to its "usability" in clinical practice (Haynes, 2001; DiCenso et al., 2009) (Fig. 3.4).

COMPUTERIZED SUPPORT SYSTEMS

At the top level of the 6S model are computerized clinical decision support systems (CCDSSs), linked to patients' electronic records. These utilize algorithms or computerized decision rules to automatically suggest an evidence-based course of action in response to information entered into the individual's record. They are designed to *aid* decision-making, in real-time, by generating automated alerts, reminders, or logic statements and/or suggestions for a course of action through linkage to evidence-based guidelines.

These systems are becoming commonplace across a variety of settings, from hospitals, to primary and community healthcare facilities, to telephone triage centers. They are well-established in medication management and are increasingly used in the management of a wide range of clinical conditions, as evidenced in systematic reviews (Bennet and Hardiker, 2017; Jia et al., 2019; Rouleau et al., 2017; Marasinghe, 2015).

GUIDELINES AND OTHER EVIDENCE SUMMARIES TO SUPPORT CLINICAL DECISION-MAKING

In the absence of CCDSSs, the next best source of information (level 2 of the model) comprises high-quality, evidence-based guidelines or other summaries of valid research evidence supporting recommendations for clinical practice.

Examples of nationally prominent repositories of evidence-based clinical practice guidelines include the following:

- The National Guideline Clearinghouse, due to be continued by ECRI Institute in Fall 2018 (https://www.ecri.org/solutions/ecri-guidelines-trust/, website users are required to log in to access the guidelines) and the Preventive Services Task Force recommendations for primary care practice (https://www.uspreventiveservicestaskforce.org/Page/Name/home)
- The Scottish Intercollegiate Guidelines Network (SIGN: www.sign.ac.uk) and the National Institute for Health and Clinical Excellence (NICE: www.nice.org.uk)
- The NHMRC (National Health and Medical Research Council) Australian Clinical Practice Guidelines (https://www.clinicalguidelines.gov.au/)
- The Canadian Medical Association Clinical Practice Guidelines Infobase (https://www.cma.ca/En/Pages/clinical-practice-guidelines.aspx)

There are also commercial evidence summary products such as *UpToDate* (https://www.uptodate.com/home/product), *DynaMed Plus* (http://www.dynamed.com/home/), and *BMJ Best Practice* (http://bestpractice.bmj.com/info/). The range of medical conditions covered by these products and the methods of evaluation used when compiling these resources vary. Libraries will advise if access to these resources has been purchased. See Chapter 8 for a more detailed discussion of guidelines.

SYNTHESES: SYSTEMATIC REVIEWS AND SYNOPSES OF SYSTEMATIC REVIEWS

In the absence of evidence-based guidelines, try to find systematic reviews or, even better, synopses of systematic reviews (levels 3 and 4 of the model).

Systematic reviews, also referred to as *secondary research*, are discussed in Chapter 7. They use explicit methods to identify, select, critically appraise, and synthesize the available research evidence pertinent to a specified question. Topic areas are diverse; for example, systematic reviews have investigated the effectiveness of interventions, accuracy of diagnostic tests, and patients' experiences of services. A major resource for systematic reviews, used to inform healthcare decision-making and policy, is *The Cochrane Library* (www.cochranelibrary.com). Databases in the library can be searched simultaneously from the opening screen (Fig. 3.5). Cochrane systematic reviews are updated at intervals to incorporate the latest research evidence and are subject to rigorous peer review.

For questions around social-oriented interventions, there is the Campbell Library, which holds a collection of systematic reviews in education, crime and justice, and social welfare. (https://www.campbellcollaboration.org/library.html).

The Joanna Briggs Institute (JBI) based at the University of Adelaide, Australia, publishes the JBI Database of Systematic Reviews and Implementation Reports, an online journal that includes healthcare-related systematic reviews created following the JBI methodology. (https://journals.lww.com/jbisrir/Pages/default.aspx).

Synopses of systematic reviews report only the essential information from the systematic reviews, and in a format that allows the reader to quickly ascertain the quality of the systematic reviews (synopses include a judgment on the quality of the systematic review) and to decide on their clinical utility, so are arguably more useful than full-text systematic reviews in a time-restricted,

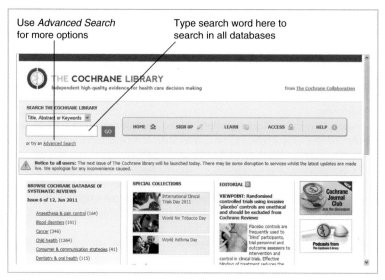

Fig. 3.5   The Cochrane Library opening screen. (Reproduced with permission from Wiley-Blackwell Ltd.)

clinical context. Examples of resources for synopses of systematic reviews include *Worldviews on Evidence-Based Nursing* (https://sigmapubs.onlinelibrary.wiley.com/journal/17416787), *Evidence-Based Nursing* (http://ebn.bmj.com/), and, for public health interventions, *Health Evidence* (https://www.healthevidence.org).

INDIVIDUAL STUDIES AND SYNOPSES OF INDIVIDUAL STUDIES

If, at this stage, no good-quality evidence has been found, then you will need to resort to individual studies, also referred to as *primary studies,* or synopses of individual studies where available (levels 5 and 6 of the model). A drawback with evidence from these levels is that it can be difficult to make sense of often contradictory results from multiple individual studies.

Staff at hospital/university libraries should be able to give advice about bibliographic databases they subscribe to, which can be searched for individual research studies (many of these databases also include guidelines, systematic reviews, and synopses). Database examples, presented in Appendix 3.1, include general biomedical databases such as CINAHL, The Cochrane Central Register of Controlled Trials (CENTRAL) within the Cochrane Library, EMBASE, and MEDLINE, and also databases with a tighter focus such as PsycINFO and PEDro.

All of these databases are produced by different organizations, so they will often look different, contain different information, and the searching tools available may vary. There will be variation between Internet and online versions of a database.

Which databases you choose to search will depend on factors such as the following:

- The specific subject of a search
- Availability
- How easy/difficult it is to search

Always make a note of which database(s) are searched, the years/date searched, the version(s), and the search terms used, for each question or project that is undertaken. This is particularly useful if the search is to be rerun in the future. It also serves as a reminder of the extent of the search.

Alternative Online Quick-Access Tools to Find Evidence

Although we have provided examples of sources of evidence for each level of the 6S model, you may find it useful to search across a number of databases simultaneously, without having to log on to each database individually.

"Search engines" such as Google are often used by healthcare professionals and patients to find information on specific diseases or interventions. However, these "generic"-type search engines produce lists of thousands of web pages, and many will not have a research focus. It is, therefore, preferable to use search engines that specifically target databases of recognized medical research publications. Google Scholar is one example. We discuss additional examples in the following sections.

TRIP (TURNING RESEARCH INTO PRACTICE) DATABASE

TRIP (http://www.tripdatabase.com/) searches a broad range of evidence-based healthcare-related websites including National Guidelines Clearinghouse (partial archive), Registered Nurses' Association of Ontario, Cochrane Library databases, the *Evidence Based Nursing* Journal, and many others. The results of the search are displayed by Category (e.g., guidelines, medical images).

SUMSEARCH 2

SUMSearch2 (http://sumsearch.org/) is hosted by the University of Kansas School of Medicine & Medical Center. When search term(s) are typed in, this system automatically checks MEDLINE and other online resources to form a collated list of results. SUMSearch 2 uses the MeSH (MEDLINE) thesaurus, so index terms and free text terms can be used to search. Search results are split into original studies, systematic reviews, and guidelines.

NHS EVIDENCE

In the UK, NHS Evidence (www.evidence.nhs.uk) provides easy access to carefully selected evidence-based resources. The search can be limited to guidelines or to systematic reviews by clicking on the appropriate filter on the search page, and results can be selected by, for example, types of information.

OTHER ONLINE COLLECTIONS

For compilations of evidence-based practice methodology, there is the "Netting the Evidence Google Search Engine" created by ScHARR (the School of Health and Related Research), at Sheffield University, which searches over 100 selected websites on EBP methods. The search engine can be found at http://tinyurl.com/2poh3a.

Healthcare bodies and professional associations, such as the American Association of Nurse Practitioners, Academy of Medical-Surgical Nurses, American College of Nurse-Midwives and the Royal College of Nursing, often flag up or give access to healthcare resources. The US Veterans Health Administration has an online medical library, the national Desktop Library, for their staff (https://www.va.gov/Library/), and the US National Library of Medicine has a portal for healthcare professionals (https://www.nlm.nih.gov/portals/healthcare.html). In the UK there is the Knowledge Network NHS Scotland (http://www.knowledge.scot.nhs.uk/home.aspx), Health on the Net Northern Ireland (HONNI) (http://www.honni.qub.ac.uk), and NHS Wales e-Library (http://www.wales.nhs.uk/researchandresources/elibrary).

BOX 3.3 ■ Key Points to Remember About Where to Search First

1. Check with your hospital or university library to identify which resources you have access to and to obtain support and advice in using them.
2. When searching for research evidence, take account of the 6S model of resources.
3. Summaries of evidence (such as evidence-based guidelines) and synopses of systematic reviews bring together all the relevant evidence in a concise and convenient package for busy clinicians to use.
4. Resort to searching for primary research articles only if more useful, "value-added" evidence (e.g., a well-conducted evidence-based guideline, a synopsis of a systematic review, or a systematic review) cannot be identified.
5. Use established bibliographic databases (organizations may have to pay for access), or use their equivalent Internet versions.
6. Use health-related "quick access" sites or links compiled by reliable groups/organizations, in preference to generic search engines, to find healthcare research.

Appendix 3.2 gives further suggestions on useful websites. Exploring the variety of evidence resources made available in your place of work is often the best place to start. Although some items may be open access, others are password-restricted. Your library staff will assist you.

Reflecting on Resources

We hope the preceding section has prompted you to take a considered approach when selecting which resources to access. Box 3.3 highlights some of the key points discussed.

An Example Search on the MEDLINE Database (PubMed Version)

This section looks at the process of undertaking a search on the MEDLINE database. MEDLINE is a general biomedical database, available in a variety of versions including PubMed, OVID, and ProQuest Dialog. We have used the PubMed version in our example. PubMed is developed by the National Center for Biotechnology Information at the US National Library of Medicine, and can be accessed free of charge at www.ncbi.nlm.nih.gov/pubmed/. PubMed provides numerous methods of searching, only some of which are described in the following sections. For further information on using this database, click on the PubMed FAQs and PubMed Tutorials links located on the home page screen (Fig. 3.6). Most healthcare databases provide detailed information on search techniques, so you should find it easy to adapt the process described in the following sections to any database.

Search terms can be entered into the Search Box of the home page (a screen shot is shown in Fig. 3.6) or the Advanced Search page accessed via the Advanced link. We prefer to work from the Advanced Search page (Fig. 3.7) as it offers more options. We use the question on needle phobia from the Basic search principles section (see Box 3.1) to build a search specifically designed for PubMed.

STEP 1: CHECKING WHAT SEARCH TOOLS ARE AVAILABLE

First check the search tools available in the database. This will usually be under the help information in the database. Check which words the database uses for Boolean logic. They are often AND, OR, and NOT. Check whether they are case-sensitive (i.e., whether you need to use

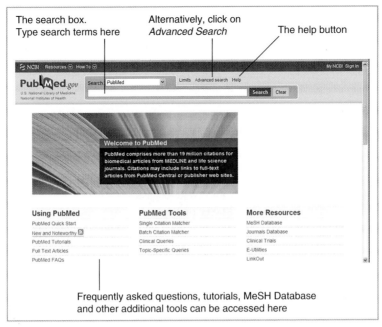

Fig. 3.6 PubMed home page. (© National Library of Medicine, reproduced with permission.)

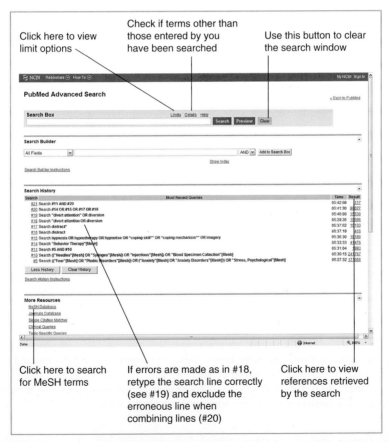

Fig. 3.7 PubMed Advanced Search page. (© National Library of Medicine, reproduced with permission.)

capital letters). Check for the symbols used for truncation and the wildcard, if available, and check whether a phrase must be specified in any way (e.g., by using quotation marks).

In PubMed, the Boolean operators are AND, OR, and NOT (uppercase); the truncation symbol is *; phrases should be enclosed in double quotes.

STEP 2: USING THE THESAURUS

Use the thesaurus to see whether there are any indexing terms that correspond to the concepts identified in your question.

The thesaurus in PubMed is known as MeSH (Medical Subject Headings). MeSH is a registered trademark of the U.S. National Library of Medicine. In PubMed, free text terms are automatically matched to appropriate MeSH (index) terms where available, provided truncation is not used. So, a search using free text terms will automatically retrieve records containing the exact typed words/phrases and records that have been assigned the relevant MeSH (index) terms. Where time restrictions call for a search with a high precision rate (i.e., with few irrelevant records), and where it is less important that all records are retrieved, then a search using index terms only (if such terms are available) can be conducted.

To view the thesaurus, click on MeSH Database link on the home page, or select under "More Resources" on the Advanced Search page, then enter a term into the Search Box to identify any corresponding MeSH terms from the thesaurus. The methods used to build a search using MeSH terms are described in Step 4.

In other databases, to view the thesaurus it may be necessary to type the search term into the search box, "turn on" a matching (mapping) facility by ticking the appropriate box, click on Search or Go, and scroll down the displayed list to find relevant index term(s). It is usually possible to click on the index term to get an exact definition/description of that term. If a useful match for a concept is found, make a note of it so it can be used in the search. Sometimes there will not be a convenient index term available, so stop searching if nothing is identified after looking up a number of different descriptions.

In addition to helping to identify index terms of interest, a thesaurus can allow searching of a group of related index terms in one go. In this example, we are interested in non-pharmacologic interventions for needle phobia. There are a number of relevant indexing terms listed in the thesaurus such as "cognitive therapy," "relaxation therapy," "meditation," and so on. Each of these terms could be added separately into a search strategy, but it would save time if all of these related indexing terms could be added in one step. This is possible in many thesauri because index terms are listed in a hierarchy.

Basic Structure of a Thesaurus

A thesaurus orders index terms into hierarchical lists, with general terms at the top and more precise, specific terms underneath. These lists are often called *tree structures* (the lists "branch out" rather like a tree). Fig. 3.8 shows a section of a thesaurus in PubMed. Terms at the top of a list are broader terms, and those indented underneath are narrower terms. In the example, "relaxation therapy" is a broader term than "meditation"; "behavior therapy" is a broader term than "relaxation therapy"; "psychotherapy" is a broader term than "behavior therapy."

Exploding Index Terms

To find articles indexed with the MeSH term "behavior therapy," and articles indexed with the narrower MeSH terms such as "relaxation therapy" and "meditation" in one step, "explode" the broader index term. PubMed defaults to the explode option, so a search of a broader term will automatically retrieve articles that have been assigned narrower MeSH terms. In other

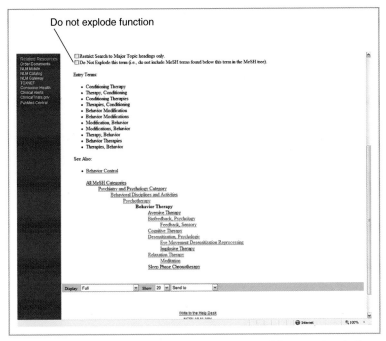

Fig. 3.8   Example of a MeSH tree in PubMed. (© National Library of Medicine, reproduced with permission.)

databases, you may need to select an "explode" button before pressing the "search" button. In PubMed, exploding the index term "behavior therapy" would automatically search the following index terms:

Behavior Therapy
    Anger Management Therapy
    Applied Behavior Analysis
    Aversive Therapy
    Biofeedback, Psychology
        Feedback, Sensory
        Neurofeedback
    Cognitive Remediation
    Cognitive Therapy
        Acceptance and Commitment Therapy
        Mindfulness
    Desensitization, Psychological
        Eye Movement Desensitization Reprocessing
        Implosive Therapy
        Virtual Reality Exposure Therapy
    Relaxation Therapy
        Meditation
    Sleep Phase Chronotherapy

The "explode" function picks up everything *beneath and indented to the right* of the exploded term. You can choose to avoid this option by activating the "Do not explode this term" button in the MeSH Database (see Fig. 3.8).

BOX 3.4 ■ Draft Search Strategy for the Question on Needle Phobia

#1   fear OR phobia OR anxiety OR stress
#2   needles OR syringes OR injections
#3   #1 AND #2
#4   cognitive behavio(u)ral therapy OR relaxation OR meditation OR meditate OR meditating
      OR desensiti(s/z)ation OR desensiti(s/z)e OR hypnosis OR hypnotherapy OR hypnotise OR
      coping skills OR relaxation
#5   distraction OR distracting OR distract OR diversion OR divert attention
#6   #4 OR #5
#7   #3 AND #6

BOX 3.5 ■ Enhanced Search Strategy for the Question on Needle Phobia*

#1   Fear OR phobic disorders OR anxiety OR anxiety disorder OR stress, psychological
#2   Needles OR syringes OR injections OR blood specimen collection
#3   #1 AND #2
#4   Behavior therapy
#5   Hypnosis OR hypnotherapy OR hypnotise OR "coping skill*" OR "coping mechanism*" OR
      imagery
#6   Distract*
#7   "Divert attention" OR diversion
#8   #4 OR #5 OR #6 OR #7
#9   #3 AND #8

---

*Designed for PubMed: MeSH terms and Boolean operators are in capital letters; phrases are
  enclosed in double quotations; and truncation (use with care) is indicated with an asterisk. Note:
  MeSH terms are used in preference to free text terms.

STEP 3: GETTING A SEARCH READY

Having checked through the details of the search tools and found some useful index terms to use, add that information into the written words/phrases list already prepared from the PICOS question. It is a good idea to have a written plan of the search terms that will be typed into the search box, and the symbols that will be used. In this way, mistakes are less likely to be made.

The search is constructed in a series of steps, each step starting on a new line. The final line of the search should bring together the combination of words you wish to find in the journal articles. Box 3.4 shows a draft, handwritten search strategy comprising free text terms that we think represent the P and I components of our needle phobia question. In Box 3.5, we have further refined the proposed search strategy to include, in places, MeSH terms as opposed to free text terms. This is to increase the precision of our search. We plan to use the exploded term "behavior therapy," which will pick up articles that have been assigned the index terms relaxation therapy, meditation, and so on (as shown in Fig. 3.8). We have, therefore, deleted free text terms such as "meditation," "meditate," "meditating," and so on.

STEP 4: ENTERING YOUR SEARCH STRATEGY ONTO THE DATABASE

At this point, the search strategy is ready to be entered. The first line of the written search strategy in the example (see Box 3.5) comprises MeSH terms that have been identified from the thesaurus. Click on the MeSH Database link (under More Resources) in the Advanced Search screen

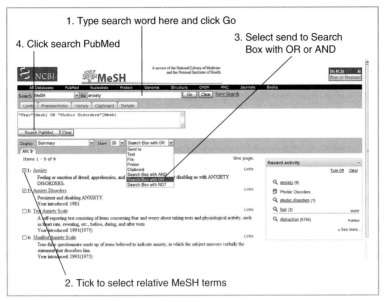

Fig. 3.9   PubMed MeSH page. (© National Library of Medicine, reproduced with permission.)

(shown in Fig. 3.7) to access the MeSH page (Fig. 3.9). Type the first term in the search box and click Search, and then select the appropriate MeSH term(s) from terms offered by ticking the relevant box(es). The default in PubMed is for the term to be exploded, so all index terms below the term selected will also be searched. Click Add to Search Builder with AND or Add to Search Builder with OR (depending on which Boolean operator is to be used), and then clear the search window (using the "x" at the end) and type the next search term to identify the MeSH term. Once all selected terms are in the search builder box, click Search PubMed. This will yield a list of references, all of which are indexed with one or more of the listed MeSH terms.

We want to add more lines from our written search to our search strategy, so we ignore this list of references and click again on the Advanced link. Continue building the search strategy: To add MeSH terms, follow the instructions described earlier; to add free text terms, type each term into the blank Builder search box, and then click Add to history. The database will look for any journal articles containing the words/phrases specified and add the results as a new line onto the History. Then enter the next search term into the automatically cleared Builder search box. In PubMed, it is possible to view exactly which terms the database has searched by looking in the Search Details box on the MeSH Database page or when viewing references. (Clicking the "See more" button underneath takes you to the full screen display Details page.) Fig. 3.10 gives a list of terms searched when the truncated term "distract*" was typed into the Builder Search Box. You can type the next line of the written search into the search box even if the Details page is open.

To view each line of the search (i.e., the search history), return to the Advanced Search page (see Fig. 3.7) by clicking the Advanced link. As shown, each line has automatically been assigned a number (#1, #2, etc.). Don't worry if, as in our search, the numbers do not start at #1 or are not consecutive. To combine the lines of the search, type the relevant line numbers and the appropriate Boolean operators into the search window, and click Add to history. Continue building the search strategy to replicate line by line (apart from the numbering) the written search plan. Fig. 3.7 shows our completed search. #21 gives the final line of the P component of the search (2722 references were identified by this part of the search); #26 gives the final line of the I component of

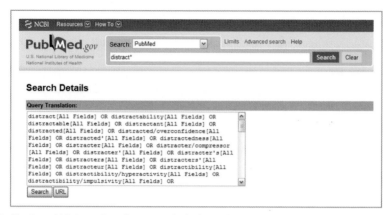

Fig. 3.10 To view which terms have been searched when using truncation, click to view the references for that search line, then click to "See more" under the Search Details box. (© National Library of Medicine, reproduced with permission.)

our search (138,995 references were identified by this part of the search). The overall final line of the search (in this example, line #27) brings together the journal articles that hopefully address the question (155 articles, some of which may be irrelevant). To view the identified references, click on the final line of the search in the Items found column (see Fig. 3.7). If you make a mistake (e.g., a spelling mistake) when searching for a term, just retype that search line, then when bringing together the lines of the search, exclude the incorrect lines.

To restrict the retrieved references to, for example, English language articles only, select the appropriate additional filters from the available options on the left of the screen. By applying filters to our search, the number of identified articles was reduced from 155 to 143. The filters applied are ticked to indicate how you have restricted the search. To remove the filters (for example, to search additional terms for which the restrictions do not apply), simply click "clear" next to the relevant filter.

Managing References

References in the final group can be viewed and selected one by one on screen; but it is often preferable to download them onto your computer, ideally using software such as EndNote or Mendeley. Software packages such as these have revolutionized the way in which bibliography lists can be generated, and references sorted and integrated into articles, dissertations, and theses. In the absence of such software, references can be saved to a file on your computer as a word document. Look for the "Send to" dropdown list to do this. There is usually the choice of which references to print/save and the specific fields to be included. In PubMed, click on the Format link to select the required format. References can be displayed as shown in Fig. 3.11 or, more helpfully, the abstracts can also be shown. Next, click the Send to link, and select File. You will then be asked where, on your computer, you would like to save the file. This completes the procedure for doing a basic search on PubMed.

Common Queries Regarding Searching

IN WHAT ORDER SHOULD SEARCH TERMS BE TYPED IN A SEARCH STRATEGY?

There are no rules on how a search should be typed out. Things can be done in any order; words/phrases can be split up so there are more lines in a search, or lumped together so there are fewer lines overall. The important thing is to ensure that the logic of each step is correct.

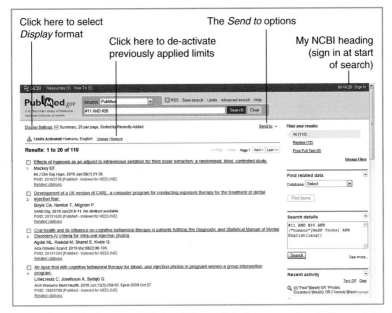

Fig. 3.11 Retrieved references. (© National Library of Medicine, reproduced with permission.)

SHOULD A SEARCH COMPRISE TERMS FROM EACH OF THE PICOS COMPONENTS?

It is advisable to search all the terms for one component of the question before starting on the next component. In this way, you will know whether or not it is necessary to add terms from a second or third component to the search. If a comprehensive list of search terms relating to the P component of your PICOS question (combined with the appropriate Boolean operator) yields the information that you need, there is no need to add search terms from other components of your PICOS question.

IS IT BETTER TO USE FREE TEXT OR CONTROLLED VOCABULARY (INDEX TERMS)?

Where index terms are available, it is advisable to use them. They limit the number of irrelevant articles identified, and overcome the need to think about all the different terms that may have been used in publications to describe an illness or population, for example. If a very thorough search is required, a combination of index terms and free text terms should be used, in case index terms have been assigned incorrectly or not assigned at all.

HOW DO YOU KNOW WHEN ALL THE RELEVANT JOURNAL ARTICLES IN A DATABASE HAVE BEEN FOUND?

There is no way to know if everything of interest has been found. Finding "most" of the useful information in a database is the best that can be hoped for. Searching is a pragmatic exercise, and there is always the possibility that something will have been missed unintentionally, regardless of the experience of the searcher.

WHAT DO YOU DO IF YOU CANNOT FIND ANY RELEVANT ARTICLES?

If you find no references at all, or items of poor quality only, it can be helpful to re-examine the question and search strategy. Devising a search strategy is a trial-and-error process, and even experienced searchers will reconsider their approach a number of times if they struggle to find any useful results. A search strategy may require a few attempts before it is finalized.

There will be occasions, however, when in spite of trying a range of strategies no high-quality information is forthcoming and the best available evidence is expert opinion.

Tips for More Advanced Users

PROXIMITY OPERATORS

Examples of proximity operators are WITH, NEAR, and ADJ, used to find words that fall in the same sentence, the same paragraph, or within a certain number of words of each other, respectively. The search "midwife WITH care team" would find articles containing at least one sentence with both midwife and care team in it, and "sickle cell NEAR leg ulcer" would find articles containing a paragraph with both sickle cell and leg ulcer in it. The search "head ADJ2 neck" would find articles containing the words head and neck within two words of each other.

Check the Help section to find out which proximity terms to use in a specific database.

LIMITING TO SPECIFIC FIELDS

Most databases allow you to search for words in a specific "field" of a journal article, such as the title or author field. In these databases, each field in an article is usually assigned an abbreviated code, which can be used when searching.

In databases where the codes TI, AU, and AB are used to identify the fields Title, Author, and Abstract, the search "injections[TI]" would find articles with the word "injections" in the title field, "Bloggs.au" would find articles with the word Bloggs in the author field, and "nurse in AB" would find articles with the word "nurse" in the abstract field. Check the Help section to identify the abbreviated codes and syntax (e.g., whether to use upper or lower case letters) for that database.

In PubMed, the search can be limited to a specific field either by adding the code (tag) using square brackets (for example, type "Bloggs[AU]" in the search box), by choosing the field from the All Fields dropdown list when using the Builder search box, or by applying the relevant Search Fields filter on the retrieved results page.

SUBHEADINGS

To help make an index term even more precise, some systems include an option to search an index term with certain subheadings attached. Subheadings are categories such as diagnosis, prevention, adverse reactions, and surgery. If it is certain that the search only needs to focus on a narrow aspect of an index term, selecting only the appropriate subheading(s) will limit the search to just the index term with that subheading attached. In PubMed, the subheadings can be viewed in the MeSH database (Fig. 3.12).

SAVING SEARCH STRATEGIES

Many database systems allow a completed search history to be saved so the search can be run again without having to type everything from scratch. In PubMed, the search history can be saved indefinitely using My NCBI. This requires that you sign into a My NCBI account before constructing the search. (Fig. 3.11 notes the My NCBI access button.) Check the Help section for more information.

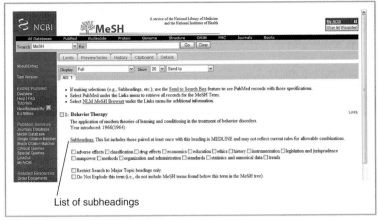

List of subheadings

Fig. 3.12 Example of a MeSH heading and its subheadings. (© National Library of Medicine, reproduced with permission.)

TOO MANY OR TOO FEW ARTICLES

If too many (irrelevant) articles are found, it may be necessary to narrow down a search to make it more specific. Use more precise index terms, or link them to selected subheadings, perhaps search over a fewer number of years, or use terms from more than one component of the PICOS question to focus down your search. Alternatively, break up a broad subject into a series of questions so the volume of information available can be better managed.

If only a few articles of interest are found, try widening the search. Use broader index terms, or more general free text terms. It is possible that a low search result could mean little research has been done on that exact topic.

WHEN TO STOP SEARCHING

This depends on the objectives of a search. If a good-quality, up-to-date evidence-based guideline or systematic review has been identified, searching may be stopped. If the objective is to identify a few articles on a topic to get an "evidence based" debate going, a quick search on one database may be quite sufficient. If a comprehensive literature review is required, a number of different databases should be searched to get as much useful material as possible (although there is over-lap between databases in journal coverage, some journals are unique to one database). However, if comprehensive searches are done on a number of different databases, there will be gradually diminishing returns. The volume of new articles identified will decrease. There will come a point when the effort involved in searching is not worth the tiny reward of new material found.

There is no right or wrong answer on when to stop searching; it is a pragmatic decision. The main thing is to be explicit about which databases have been searched. This avoids any confusion and allows a search to be accurately updated or expanded by looking in different databases.

Searching for a Systematic Review

Teaching the searching skills for a systematic review is beyond the scope of this manual, but help can be sought from specialist librarians or information specialists. A systematic review entails an exhaustive search of databases and other resources to try to identify as many relevant ongoing and completed studies as possible. This requires searching experience. Budgeting is necessary to ensure all searching-related activities (building comprehensive search strategies, accessing the appropriate databases, identifying hard-to-find studies, obtaining and translating articles) can be completed within the funding limitations.

Some published research can be difficult to find: unexpected terminology may have been used; articles may not have been assigned index terms; not all good-quality research work is published in professional journals; much research is published in the form of conference proceedings, theses, or project reports only; many journals are not included in electronic databases. Systematic reviewers are charged with tracking down not only the easily accessible research, but also these more difficult to find studies.

The Cochrane Collaboration has a commitment to try and locate hard to find RCTs by searching conference proceedings and by looking through journals by hand ("hand searching"). Any extra RCTs found in this way are published in the Cochrane Central Register of Controlled Trials on the Cochrane Library. This means that searching this database on the Cochrane Library provides a practical solution for finding information for systematic reviews focusing on the effectiveness of interventions (the RCT is the optimum study design to address effectiveness questions).

Much work is being done to encourage researchers to publish their research proposals. This has enabled systematic reviewers to identify research that is in progress, or completed but not yet published. Major resources for clinical research in progress are ClinicalTrials.gov from the US National Institutes of Health (https://clinicaltrials.gov) and the ISCRTN registry (https://www.isrctn.com/), and the UK Clinical trials Gateway (https://www.ukctg.nihr.ac.uk/clinical-trials/search-for-a-clinical-trial/) can be used to search both these resources.

USEFUL GUIDES FOR SYSTEMATIC REVIEWERS

- Centre for Reviews and Dissemination. *Systematic Reviews: CRD's Guidance for undertaking systematic reviews in healthcare,* 3rd edition, 2009. Chapter 1, Section 1.3.1.: Identifying research evidence for systematic reviews; Appendix 2: Example search strategy to identify studies from electronic databases (https://www.york.ac.uk/crd/guidance/)
- Lefebvre C, Manheimer E, Glanville J. Chapter 6: Searching for studies. In: Higgins JPT, Green S (eds). *Cochrane Handbook for Systematic Reviews of Interventions* Version 5.1.0 (updated March 2011). The Cochrane Collaboration, 2011 (www.handbook.cochrane.com)
- de Vet HCW, Eisinga A, Riphagen II, Aertgeerts B, Pewsner D. Chapter 7: Searching for Studies. In: Cochrane Handbook for Systematic Reviews of Diagnostic Test Accuracy Version 0.4 (updated September 2008). The Cochrane Collaboration, 2008 (http://methods.cochrane.org/sdt/handbook-dta-reviews)

Practicing Your Search Skills

We hope the preceding sections have outlined the benefits of using a systematic approach when searching electronic databases. Box 3.6 is an aide memoir for the various aspects of searching that you may want to practice. We encourage you undertake the online exercises available at http://evolve.elsevier.com/Craig/evidence/

Summary

This chapter has provided an introduction on how to search the research literature to support evidence-based practice in health care. It has provided background on how databases of individual articles are organized and the basic principles that are used when searching for information on electronic systems. The use of the 6S model for selecting resources to search has been highlighted.

BOX 3.6 ■ Key Points to Remember About Searching Electronic Databases

1. Get help.
   Attend training sessions in hospital/university libraries. Find out about support for searching in general.
2. Prepare the search.
   Sort out the question/topic, generate word lists, have a draft search planned.
3. Find out more.
   What database(s) might be useful to search, what tools they have (e.g., truncation, thesaurus), and how these tools are used. Check the "help" information and any written guidelines.
4. Decide which database to search.
   Plan so that you search resources in order of usefulness. Do a brief test search, check ease of searching, and make sure all useful information is available.
5. Prepare the final search strategy.
   Add in index terms, truncation symbols, and so on for the database to be searched.
6. Do the search.
   Select index terms; type in free text terms. Get the final set of useful records at the end.
7. Print or save the final set of articles.
   Print/save the records to look at later.
8. Keep a record of the resources searched.
   Make a note of the database, the version used (e.g., Ovid online, ProQuest Dialog online), the years searched, and the date the search was done.
9. Keep a record of the search strategy.
   Make sure a copy is kept, so the exact details are available for future reference.
10. If searching for systematic review, access sources of unpublished and ongoing research.

An example search on PubMed and some discussion of more advanced searching techniques has also been covered. The resources that are available to search will depend on local funding and access arrangements, so the importance of consulting the library services of which you are a member has been emphasized. Your library should be the first port of call to assist with searching questions and to provide hands-on training sessions and individual support on the resources it provides. It may also be able to undertake searches for research evidence on your behalf.

References

Bennett, P., Hardiker, N.R., 2017. The use of computerized clinical decision support systems in emergency care: a substantive review of the literature. J. Am. Med. Inform. Assoc. 24 (3), 655–668.

DiCenso, A., Bayley, L., Haynes, B., 2009. Accessing pre-appraised evidence: fine-tuning the 5S model into a 6S model. Evid. Based Nurs. 12 (4), 99–101.

Haynes, R.B., 2001. Of studies, syntheses, synopses and systems: the "4S" evolution of services for finding current best evidence. Evid. Based Med. 6 (2), 36–38.

Jia, P., Zhao, P., Chen, J., Zhang, M., 2019. Evaluation of clinical decision support systems for diabetes care: an overview of current evidence. J. Eval. Clin. Pract. 25 (1), 66–77. https://doi.org/10.1111/jep.12968. [Epub 2018 Jun 26].

Marasinghe, K.M., 2015. Computerised clinical decision support systems to improve medication safety in long-term care homes: a systematic review. BMJ Open 5 (5), e006539.

Centre for Reviews and Dissemination, 2009. Systematic reviews. CRD's guidance for undertaking reviews in healthcare. 3rd Edition. Available from https://www.york.ac.uk/crd/guidance/ (Accessed 20.04.19.).

Rouleau, G., Gagnon, M.-P., Côté, J., Payne-Gagnon, J., Hudson, E., Dubois, C.-A., 2017. Impact of information and communication technologies on nursing care: results of an overview of systematic reviews. J. Med. Internet Res. 19 (4), e122.

Further Reading

These are general articles about searching the healthcare literature aimed at the beginner/intermediate. As far as possible, they are directed at a nursing audience. Some older references, which remain relevant, have been included in the list.

Aromataris, E., Riitano, D., 2014. Systematic reviews: constructing a search strategy and searching for evidence. Am. J. Nurs. 14 (5), 49–56.

Considine, J., Shaban, R.Z., Fry, M., Curtis, K., 2017. Evidence based emergency nursing: designing a research question and searching the literature. Int. Emerg. Nurs. 32, 78–82.

Facchinano, L., Snyder, C.H., 2012. Evidence-based practice for the busy nurse practitioner: part two: searching for the evidence to clinical enquiries. J. Am. Acad. Nurse Prac. 24 (11), 640–648.

Lawrence, J.C., 2007. Techniques for searching the CINAHL database using the EBSCO interface. AORN J 85 (4), 779–791.

National Health Service Centre for Reviews and Dissemination Centre for Reviews and Dissemination, 2001. Accessing the evidence on clinical effectiveness. Effectiveness Matters 5 (1) . Available from: https://www.york.ac.uk/media/crd/em51.pdf (Accessed 20.04.19.).

Robb, M., Shellenbarger, T., 2014. Strategies for searching and managing evidence-based practice resources. J. Contin. Educ. Nurs. 45 (10), 461–466.

Waltho, D., Kaur, M.N., Haynes, R.B., Farrokhyar, F., Thoma, A., 2015. Users' guide to the surgical literature: how to perform a high-quality literature search. Can. J. Surg. 58 (5), 349–358.

Windish, D., 2013. Searching for the right evidence: how to answer your clinical questions using the 6S hierarchy. Evid. Based Med. 18 (3), 93–97.

Young, J.S., 2010. PubMed searching for home clinicians: a guide for success in identifying articles for a literature review. Home Healthc. Nurse 28 (9), 559–565.

Appendix 3.1 Bibliographic Databases (Collections of Research Articles)

This is by no means a comprehensive list, but it illustrates a range of databases, some of which may be available via hospitals or universities. For additional examples, see the Cochrane Handbook for Systematic Reviews of Interventions (Chapter on searching), available at http://training.cochrane.org/handbook.

General
CINAHL

Cumulative Index to Nursing and Allied Health Literature, produced by the publisher EBSCO. Uses index terms and has a thesaurus (called the Subject Heading List).
British Nursing Database (formerly British Nursing Index)
Produced in the UK. Contains information on nursing and midwifery, including full-text.
EMBASE
Produced by the publisher Elsevier. Uses index terms and has a thesaurus (known as Emtree).
MEDLINE/PubMed
Produced by the US National Library of Medicine (NLM). There are a number of versions available. PubMed is the free Internet version. Uses index terms and has a thesaurus (MeSH).
Specialist
AgeLine
Produced by EBSCO. Covers issues of aging and the population aged 50 years and older. Uses index terms and has a thesaurus (AgeLine's Thesaurus of Aging Terminology).

AIDSLINE

Database of information on HIV and AIDS, produced by the NLM.

AMED

Allied and Complementary Medicine, produced by the British Library. Includes physiotherapy, occupational therapy, rehabilitation, and palliative care. Uses index terms and has a thesaurus (AMED thesaurus, based on MeSH).

CABHealth

Database of information relating to human nutrition; parasitic, communicable (including AIDS/HIV), and tropical diseases; medicinal plants; and public health. Strong international and developing country coverage. Uses index terms and has a thesaurus (CAB thesaurus).

CANCERLIT

Database of information on cancer, produced by the US National Cancer Institute.

HMIC

Health Management Information Consortium database. Produced in the UK, an amalgamation of databases from the Nuffield Institute of Health (University of Leeds), the Department of Health, and the King's Fund.

LLBA

Linguistics and Language Behavior Abstracts. Coverage includes speech, language, and hearing pathology.

PEDro

Physiotherapy evidence database.

PsycINFO

Produced by the American Psychological Association. Covers all aspects of psychology. Uses index terms and has a thesaurus (Thesaurus of Psychological Index Terms) for items dating from 1967 onward.

Others

EVIDENCE BASED MEDICINE REVIEWS

This combines a selection of renowned evidence-based resources, such as the following resources, into one database:

1. The Cochrane Library, which includes databases of systematic reviews and also the Cochrane Central Register of Controlled Trials (CENTRAL), a comprehensive bibliographic database of randomized controlled trials and controlled clinical trials in health care that is an excellent source of evidence for questions about effectiveness of an intervention or investigation in the absence of a systematic review.
2. *The American College of Physicians (ACP) Journal Club journal.*
3. *Evidence Based Medicine.*

SCIENCE CITATION INDEX

An electronic version of the *Current Contents* publications covering scientific journals. Aims to add newly published articles on to the database promptly.

Social Science Citation Index

Sister publication to Science Citation Index, covering social science journals.

Appendix 3.2 Useful Websites

NURSING ORGANIZATIONS

American Association of Nurse Practitioners: www.aanp.org

American College of Nurse-Midwives: www.midwife.org

American Nurses Association: www.nursingworld.org

Australian College of Nursing: www.acn.edu.au

Canadian Nurses Association: www.cna-aiic.ca/en

Midwives Information and Resource Service (MIDIRS), a "not-for-profit" charity: www.midirs.org/

Royal College of Nursing: www.rcn.org.uk

Royal College of Midwives: www.rcm.org.uk/

EVIDENCE-BASED PRACTICE ORGANIZATIONS

AHRQ Evidence-Based Practice Centers Evidence-Based Reports: www.ahrq.gov/research/findings/evidence-based-reports/index.html

Campbell Collaboration: www.campbellcollaboration.org/

Campbell Collaboration databases library: www.campbellcollaboration.org/library.html

CareSearch (Palliative Care Knowledge Network, Australia): https://www.caresearch.com.au/caresearch/tabid/80/Default.aspx

Cochrane Collaboration: www.cochrane.org/

Cochrane Library: cochranelibrary.com

Cochrane Library User Guide: www.cochranelibrary.com/help/how-to-use

Cochrane US Center: http://us.cochrane.org/about-us

EPPI-Centre, UK based (focused on areas of social policy including, health, social care and education): https://eppi.ioe.ac.uk/cms/

Helene Fuld Health Trust National Institute for Evidence-Based Practice in Nursing and Healthcare (Ohio State University): https://ctep-ebp.com

Joanna Briggs Institute (Australia): joannabriggs.org

NHS Centre for Reviews and Dissemination (includes the publication Effectiveness Matters): www.york.ac.uk/inst/crd/

HEALTHCARE GUIDANCE AND GUIDELINES

CMA Clinical Practice Guidelines Infobase: www.cma.ca/En/Pages/clinical-practice-guidelines.aspx

National Guideline Clearinghouse (US guidelines) due to be continued by ECRI Institute in Fall 2018: https://www.ecri.org/solutions/ecri-guidelines-trust/

National Institute for Health and Clinical Excellence (NICE): www.nice.org.uk

NHMRC Australian Clinical Practice Guidelines: www.clinicalguidelines.gov.au

NICE CKS (Clinical Knowledge Summaries): https://cks.nice.org.uk/

Scottish Intercollegiate Guidelines Network (available in the UK): www.sign.ac.uk

US Preventive Services Task Force, recommendations for primary care practice: www.uspreventiveservicestaskforce.org/Page/Name/home

CHAPTER 4

Using Evidence from Qualitative Studies

Bernie Carter ■ Helena Dunbar

KEY POINTS

- Qualitative research is fundamentally interpretative, illuminating subjective meanings and committed to the expansion of knowledge through the partnership of the researcher and the participants.
- Qualitative research encompasses a range of different theoretical and methodological frameworks.
- Qualitative research is based on the collection of word/text/language and image-based data.
- Critical appraisal requires knowledge of different methodologies and methods and being able to make connections between the approaches used and claims made within a paper.
- Qualitative research can independently contribute to evidence as well as enhance quantitative research.

Introduction

This chapter focuses on qualitative research, its contribution to evidence-based practice, and how to appraise and use evidence from qualitative studies. Although rooted in social science, qualitative research is now firmly established within nursing (Kornhaber et al., 2015) and other healthcare research. Indeed, as Porter (2010, p. 495) notes there is "compelling evidence that qualitatively generated knowledge is an essential component to the development and application of optimal care."

The term *qualitative research* encompasses a sometimes baffling (Creswell and Poth, 2018) and diverse range of different research methodologies and, as such, it can be difficult to define. However, it can broadly be described as:

> "…. the methodological pursuit of understanding the ways that people see, view, approach, and experience the world and make meaning of their experiences as well as specific phenomena within it"
> (RAVITCH AND MITTTENFELNER, 2016, p. 7).

It is the concern with making the "world of the individual visible to the rest of us" (Lobiondo-Wood and Haber, 2018, p. 89) that means that qualitative research contributes in a distinctive manner to the development of evidence and the development of practice.

Examples of the types of questions that qualitative research can explore include questions that aim to understand people's experiences of illness or treatments, their views on barriers and/or facilitators to engagement with health services or treatments, and reasons why an intervention does or does not work.

Qualitative research is sometimes described in terms of how it differs from quantitative research. Although this portrayal can be a helpful introduction to the research landscape, it may give the impression that research is composed of just two entities: quantitative (solely focused on measurement) versus qualitative (solely focused on narrative, meanings, and social experience). The reality is that both quantitative and qualitative research encompass a wide range of approaches.

Traditionally, evidence from quantitative study designs such as randomized controlled trials and systematic reviews of randomized controlled trials has been preferenced by decision makers, with qualitative research all too often being relegated to a lowly position and "rendered invisible" (Pearson, 2010, p. 489). However, there is now increasing recognition that qualitative evidence, used either on its own or in combination with quantitative evidence (such as in the case of mixed methods research, discussed in Chapter 6), can present a deeper and more complete knowledge base upon which to deliver health care. Qualitative evidence has a growing role in decision-making (Lewin et al., 2018a) and is considered a "strong and necessary contributor to health care research" (Lau et al., 2017, p. 332). Its contribution to evidence-based practice is extensive (Box 4.1). In being able to represent the views and experiences of a wide range of stakeholders (patients, families, carers, healthcare providers, managers, the wider public), it promotes an evidence base that is democratic and publicly accountable (Lewin et al., 2018a).

Used as standalone evidence, qualitative research findings that are derived from meta-synthesis (which can be defined as the interpretive integration of findings from a number of qualitative studies) can be particularly useful (Coffey et al., 2016; Webster et al., 2015). When undertaken in tandem with quantitative research, qualitative research can bring much-needed insights to the findings of the quantitative research. Increasingly there is a sense that qualitative research has value in informing the evidence base surrounding complex interventions (Cooper et al., 2014; Farquhar et al., 2011). Detailed qualitative investigation can help to provide possible reasons as to why the complex intervention, such as a behavioral change intervention, did or did not work, providing a deeper understanding of the study findings.

In this chapter, we examine the common characteristics and attributes of qualitative research. We overview different theoretical perspectives, methodologies, and methods used within qualitative research and explore the way that these, and the type of questions researchers ask, frame the

---

BOX 4.1 ■ Potential Contributions of Qualitative Research to Evidence-Based Practice

- Contribute a more complex, nuanced, and meaning-oriented understanding of the health experiences of stakeholders (van Wijngaarden et al., 2017)
- Contribute to randomized controlled trials (Audrey, 2011)
- Inform evidence base for therapeutic decision-making (La Caze, 2016)
- Illuminate the context (Kozleski, 2017)
- Contribute to decision-making by representing stakeholders' perspectives (Lewin et al., 2018a)
- Contribute to development of guidelines (Lewin et al., 2018b)
- Contribute evidence to guide holistic practice (Porter et al., 2012)
- Contribute to policy decisions in health and social care (Toews et al., 2017)
- Inform decision-making about use of evidence-based interventions (Toews et al., 2017)
- Contribute a range of evidence that goes beyond the "rationalist" model of systematic reviews that rely solely on quantitative research (Tong et al., 2012)
- Open up new avenues of discovery that had not been expected at the conception of the study (Lobiondo-Wood and Haber, 2018)
- May provide the first systematic insights into aspects of care that are not well understood (Lobiondo-Wood and Haber, 2018)

research studies they carry out. We then examine some of the different approaches to appraising qualitative research. In particular, we consider two of the most commonly used checklists that are used to guide appraisal of qualitative research, and examine topic areas that are commonly addressed in appraisal checklists.

Characteristics of Qualitative Research

There are many different ways of describing qualitative research as it encompasses a range of different theoretical and methodological frameworks. This complexity has arisen, in part, because qualitative research has evolved within a number of different disciplines such as anthropology, sociology, psychology, and nursing, each of which has contributed to its development and shaped the way that it is presented. Furthermore, undertaking research with human beings about their lives is complicated (Roller and Lavrakas, 2015). Qualitative research embraces the complexities of human realities and the intricacies of human thought and behavior (Roller and Lavrakas, 2015), and focuses on trying to generate descriptions and contextually rich interpretations of particular phenomena. It is therefore by necessity "explanatory, descriptive and inductive in nature" (Toles and Barros, 2018, p. 89). One way of trying to understand qualitative research is to draw on Stake's (2010, pp. 15–16) six special characteristics of qualitative study:

1. *Interpretive.* Qualitative research is predicated on the belief that people perceive things in their own ways, attribute their individual meanings to things, and construct meaning based on their unique understanding of situations and what is at stake. Qualitative research therefore accepts the notion of multiple realities or multiple points of view.

2. *Experiential and field oriented;* another term used to describe this is *naturalistic.* In this sense, qualitative research is carried out in a natural setting that is (usually) not manipulated (often described as the "field") to try and explore how behaviors, experiences, and opinions are expressed in the everyday world.

3. *Situational* and orientated to *context.* This links to points 1 and 2 above, but extends to the ways in which qualitative researchers accept that life (and research), and the way we respond to situations is influenced by the things that surround us and by our prior experiences; and that these influences need to be taken into account if we are to understand them. The uniqueness of a particular setting and participants is thus highly relevant. The importance of context and the situational nature of qualitative research means that it is rare that it is designed to be generalizable, although good qualitative research aims to resonate with other situations, settings, and experiences that have similarity to the one described.

4. *Personalistic.* Researchers value people's world views, aiming to understand individual perceptions. By "following the data," laying aside their own perspective or personal values, and adopting an emic perspective (which considers "the concerns and values recognized in the behavior and language of the people being studied" [Stake, 2010, p. 55]), the researcher aims to understand issues of importance to the participants rather than those that researcher(s) might see as important.

5. *Well triangulated, well informed and reflexive.* Because qualitative research relies on interpretation, these interpretations need to be robust and built on solid data that the researcher has interrogated for alternative explanations. There are different types of triangulation (e.g., theoretical, methodological, methods, cases, investigator, data) but the basic principle underlying triangulation is to draw a conclusion from more than one source or perspective. A well-reported study provides the reader with enough information to draw his or her own conclusions. Through the use of *reflexivity* (critical self-reflection) within the study, and in the reporting of the study, the researcher's own particular position and other factors that could have influenced interpretation should be made clear.

6. Influenced by ***strategic choices.*** Some choices are made at the start of the study and are guided by its underpinning purpose, for example, choices about the purpose of the study (whether it is to contribute to policy development or to develop an in-depth understanding of individual experiences). Other choices are made as the study progresses, for example, the question asked in an interview, or the people included in the sample.

Beyond these six characteristics, qualitative research can be described pragmatically, in terms of the data it aims to collect (mostly narrative text/word and/or image based but not numerical data), the methods it uses to collect data (e.g., interviews, focus groups, diaries, photographs, observing), and how it goes about analyzing these data (e.g., through interpretation). It can also be categorized in accordance with the philosophical stance adopted by the researcher in framing their research question and how this then influences their approach to answering that question. The different approaches are informed by the researchers' beliefs about what exists and what constitutes social reality (Blaikie, 2010). Good qualitative research is generally a combination of clear and consistent philosophical decisions and choices about how to generate and analyze the data.

Appraising Qualitative Studies

Central to critical appraisal is the process of asking appropriate questions of a published research study, to elicit the extent to which the findings of that study are likely to be trustworthy and useful in a particular circumstance or setting. Finding answers to these questions in studies that are poorly described can be difficult. Thankfully, the reporting of studies has improved markedly in the last decade due to journal editors' insistence that articles must meet a minimum set of reporting standards to be accepted for publication. COREQ (consolidated criteria for reporting qualitative research), developed by Tong et al. (2007) is one example of a standard for reporting, and is a useful learning resource for novice qualitative researchers.

CRITICAL APPRAISAL CHECKLISTS

Seminal work by Lincoln and Guba (1985) proposed four criteria that still guide many readers when establishing whether or not a study is sound (Table 4.1).

Subsequently, many checklists have been developed with the aim of helping readers appraise qualitative research. However, there is no clear consensus about what criteria (or questions) should be included, or what weighting, if any, should be ascribed to the criteria. The sheer volume and variety of these checklists, and the "discrepancies both in vocabulary and in structure" (Santiago-Delefosse et al., 2016, p. 151) means that choosing the right one can feel overwhelming.

TABLE 4.1 ■ Criteria for Judging the Trustworthiness of Qualitative Studies

Criteria	Meaning
Credibility	The extent to which the findings are credible
Transferability	The extent to which the findings can be transferred to another context
Dependability	The extent to which the findings can be repeated with the same or similar subjects in the same or similar context
Confirmability	The degree to which the findings are determined by the participants and not by the biases, motivations, or perspectives of the researcher

From Lincoln, Y.S., Guba, E.G., 1985. Naturalistic Inquiry. Sage Publications: Newbury Park.

A brief glance at the critical appraisal criteria proposed in two different publications gives a feel for this diversity. Tracy (2010) proposes 8 "big tent" criteria for the consideration of "excellent" qualitative research, these being: worthy topic, rich rigor, sincerity, credibility, resonance, significant contribution, ethical, and meaningful coherence. In contrast, Roller and Lavrakas (2015) propose the total quality framework, which is based on four interrelated elements: credibility, analyzability, transparency, and usefulness (Roller and Lavrakas, 2015, p. 363).

Santiago-Delefosse et al. (2016) analyzed 58 quality assessment checklists or guidelines and identified 12 essential criteria and associated *broad* definitions that their expert group could agree upon: theoretical framework; research question; goals and objectives; literature (review); methodology/method/design; sampling; data; analysis; reflexivity; credibility; transferability; and ethics (Santiago-Delefosse et al., 2016, p. 144). However, it was clear from their work that different disciplinary groups assigned different weight to the criteria and there was less consensus in terms of the actual specific detail within the broad definitions. They conclude that future work should "promote a flexible list of criteria, that is, a 'toolbox' meeting the needs and specificities of different research" (Santiago-Delefosse et al., 2016, p. 151). This view chimes with Cohen and Crabtree's (2006) assertion that there cannot and should not be one set of criteria used to evaluate qualitative research.

There is considerable merit in the notion of approaching appraisal using a flexible toolbox approach. However, in order to effectively use a flexible toolbox, the appraiser needs to have a robust knowledge of qualitative research to make the appropriate decisions. In comparison, a "fixed" pre-prescribed checklist offers a more accessible starting point for appraisers with less experience of qualitative research.

Two examples of such checklists are the Critical Appraisal Skills Programme (CASP) checklist for qualitative research (https://casp-uk.net/aboutus/) and the Joanna Briggs Institute (JBI) checklist for qualitative research (http://joannabriggs.org). These are generic tools for use with any qualitative study, regardless of the methodology used. They can be applied to ethnographic, phenomenologic, or any other qualitative studies. Although this is a strength, a related weakness is that generic checklists cannot illuminate the nuances of what an appraiser should be considering within a particular qualitative research methodology.

The CASP Checklist for Qualitative Research

The CASP checklist for qualitative research considers three broad issues and asks 10 specific questions (Box 4.2). The appraiser has the option to choose from three responses to the questions (yes, no, can't tell), and hints are provided within the form to guide the appraiser to make an appropriate decision. Space is provided after each question for the appraiser to make comments. The first two questions act as screening questions; if the answers to these questions is "no," it is not deemed to be worth continuing to review the rest of the paper.

It is clear in the guidance notes that the checklist was designed to be used as an "educational pedagogic tool" (CASP, qualitative checklist). Although this tool is clearly useful, it has the potential to oversimplify "what stands for quality in qualitative research" (Chenail, 2011, p. 246) and to be "less sensitive to aspects of validity" than tools such as the JBI checklist.

The JBI Checklist for Qualitative Research

The JBI checklist for qualitative research, which we have used in our exemplar appraisal of a paper (see http://evolve.elsevier.com/Craig/evidence/), was designed for use in systematic reviews (see Box 4.2). It is composed of 10 questions. The appraiser has the option to choose from four responses to the questions (yes, no, unclear, not applicable) and guidance notes are provided within the form to guide the appraiser to make an appropriate decision. There are no screening questions, space is provided at the end of the form for comments, and there is a requirement to make an overall appraisal decision (include, exclude, seek further information). The guidance seems to

---

BOX 4.2 ■ Content of CASP and JBI Checklists for Appraising Qualitative Research

CASP

Section A: Are the Results of the Study Valid?

1. Was there a clear statement of the aims of the research?
2. Is a qualitative methodology appropriate?
3. Was the research design appropriate to address the aims of the research?
4. Was the recruitment strategy appropriate to the aims of the research?
5. Was the data collected in a way that addressed the research issue?
6. Has the relationship between researcher and participants been adequately considered?

Section B: What are the Results?

7. Have ethical issues been taken into consideration?
8. Was the data analysis sufficiently rigorous?
9. Is there a clear statement of findings?

Section C: Will the Results Help Locally?

10. How valuable is the research?

JBI

1. Is there congruity between the stated philosophical perspective and the research methodology?
2. Is there congruity between the research methodology and the research question or objectives?
3. Is there congruity between the research methodology and the methods used to collect data?
4. Is there congruity between the research methodology and the representation and analysis of data?
5. Is there a statement locating the researcher culturally or theoretically?
6. Is the influence of the researcher on the research, and vice versa, addressed?
7. Is there congruity between the research methodology and the interpretation of results?
8. Are participants, and their voices, adequately represented?
9. Is the research ethical according to current criteria or, for recent studies, and is there evidence of ethical approval by an appropriate body?
10. Do the conclusions drawn in the research report flow from the analysis, or interpretation, of the data?

From Critical Appraisal Skills Programme, 2018. CASP Qualitative Checklist. Available from: https://casp-uk.net/casp-tools-checklists/ (Accessed 12.11.18.).

---

assume a higher level of knowledge about qualitative research than the CASP tool. The focus of the first five questions in the JBI tool are on congruity, defined here as each element of a qualitative study fitting appropriately with other elements, and which Hannes et al. (2010) propose makes the tool more coherent as a qualitative appraisal tool than CASP.

The appraisal of qualitative work is contentious. There is a strong pull from the evidence-based healthcare communities for a checklist that can effectively facilitate appraisal of quality, and a strong resistance by some researchers who perceive checklists to be reductionist, resulting in only assessing the easier-to-reach components of a qualitative study.

SO, ARE CHECKLISTS THE ANSWER?

It is worth bearing in mind that checklists are simply a means of checking key components. They rely on the appraiser being appropriately knowledgeable about the relevant philosophical/theoretical and methodological underpinnings of a study to be able to make sensible choices about their responses. For example, some basic understanding of the theoretical underpinning of phenomenology is needed to critically appraise a phenomenological study. Although checklists generally include prompts or hints, these will make little sense to an appraiser without sufficient knowledge of qualitative research methodology, its methods, and so on.

Drawing on the work by Santiago-Delefosse et al. (2016) and the CASP and JBI tools, we have identified a set of core knowledge domains that anyone appraising qualitative research needs to understand in order to effectively use his or her selected critical appraisal checklist. We discuss each domain and highlight the key issues the appraiser needs to consider when appraising a qualitative study.

Core Knowledge Domains for Critical Appraisal

RESEARCH QUESTION, AIMS, GOALS, AND OBJECTIVES

The starting point for an appraisal is the research question and/or aim(s)/purpose/intention and goals/objectives of the study. You need to determine whether a qualitative approach was appropriate to answer the specific research question and whether the researchers have provided a clear rationale for its use. You should be able to identify a clearly articulated research question and/or aim to judge if the qualitative approach is relevant. For example, if the aim of a study was "to measure the impact on the quality of life of an intervention based on motivational interviewing for people with chronic pain, at six months from baseline, compared with conventional treatment" you would question the relevance of using a qualitative approach. Alternatively, if the stated aim was "to develop an understanding of the experiences of people with chronic pain who have received motivational interviewing," then you would have more confidence that a qualitative approach was appropriate.

PHILOSOPHICAL PERSPECTIVE

The philosophical perspective relates to the beliefs and ideas that underpin the research (Creswell and Poth, 2018) and the assumptions that are associated with them. The philosophical perspective adopted by the researchers will have implications for every stage of the research process. The choice of philosophical perspective is strongly linked to the assumptions held by the researcher. Different theoretical perspectives (sometimes called *interpretive paradigms* or *frameworks*) exist, for example, social constructivism (interpretivism), transformative frameworks, pragmatism, feminism, critical theory, and queer theory. Each perspective adopts different positions or values in terms of the stance it takes in relation to reality, for example, feminist research is often underpinned by emancipatory values, pragmatism is more concerned with finding solutions to problems, and queer theory shuns normalization. These positions and values affect the way that knowledge is created and the focus of research (Box 4.3), as well as the approach taken to appraise the study.

Knowing what theoretical/interpretive perspective/paradigm/framework informed the study enables you to make the right connections and question, for example, whether a study that claimed to use a transformative framework did actually try to challenge influences and bring about change or whether one that aimed to adopt a feminist perspective was appropriately collaborative and non-exploitative.

METHODOLOGY/APPROACH

The term *methodology* refers to the specific framework chosen by the researchers to underpin and frame their research. It provides the researcher with a structure for how to do his or her study, and among other things, guides his or her choice of methods and analytical approach (Schwandt, 2015). Different research questions and problems lend themselves to particular methodologies; the choice is guided by the nature of the initial research question. Creswell and Poth (2018) suggest that the

---

BOX 4.3 ▪ Example of Commonly Adopted Theoretical/Interpretive Perspectives

- *Social constructivism/interpretivism* focuses on understanding the world through exploring partici-pants' views of a situation and in trying to "generate or inductively develop a theory or pattern of meaning" to explain the subjective meanings of individuals' experiences (Creswell and Poth 2018, p. 24).
- *Transformative frameworks* aim to be more radical than social constructivism, and they explore and challenge how social, political, cultural, economic, or ethnic influences become integrated into social structures and influence experiences, behavior, and beliefs. A central tenet of transformative frameworks is that "knowledge is not neutral and it reflects the power and social relationships within society" (Creswell and Poth, 2018, p. 25). The aim of transformative research is to address issues such as oppression and to improve society.
- *Pragmatism* views "knowledge as an instrument or tool for organizing experience and it is deeply concerned with the union of theory and practice" (Schwandt, 2015) and focuses on questions about "what works."
- *Feminism* covers a diverse range of different theoretical perspectives that "reflect the changes in thinking about feminism, and shifts in socio-political preoccupations" (Griffin, 2017). Feminism centers on and problematizes "women's diverse situations and the institutions that frame those situ-ations" (Creswell and Poth, 2018, p. 27). It is broadly emancipatory and transformative in nature and challenges dominant assumptions relating to women.
- *Critical theory* subjects the "taken-for-granted character of the social world......to critical recon-sideration and is this part of the self-reflective public discourse of a democratic society" (Schwandt 2015). It is concerned with "empowering human beings to transcend the constraints placed on them by race, class, and gender" (Creswell and Poth, 2018, p. 27).
- *Queer theory* covers a range of different perspectives exploring the "myriad complexities of the construct, identity, and how identities reproduce and "perform" in social forums (Creswell and Poth, 2018, p. 30) and is noted to be "notoriously difficult to define" but "at a minimum queer theory challenges understandings of gender and sexuality as singular and stable" (Richter-Montpetit 2018, p. 224).

---

five main approaches are grounded theory, narrative inquiry/research, phenomenological research, ethnographic research, and case study research. However, other approaches/methodologies exist, and these include participatory research, action research, and appreciative inquiry (Box 4.4).

When appraising a paper, you need to look to see if there is a clear statement about the methodology/approach. Knowing whether the study adopted a narrative or ethnographic or phe-nomenological approach is crucial to the process of critical appraisal, as this should determine the questions you might ask. For example, an appreciative inquiry study that did not engage col-laboratively with participants, and focused solely on the problems in the study setting, would be at odds with the appreciative purpose of the study.

METHODS OF DATA COLLECTION AND SOURCES OF DATA

The most common methods of data collection used in qualitative research can be divided into four categories based around observation, verbal methods, visual methods, and existing documents and materials (Box 4.5). These methods are used to generate rich, in-depth, context-rich data. The key focus of your attention in appraising this element of a study should be on their relevance to the research question and methodological framework, and the clarity and level of detail with which the methods are described. The most commonly used methods are interviews, focus groups, and observation, although visual methods are increasing in prominence. Researchers can sometimes be tempted to use a method simply because it is appealing or innovative, rather than it being a good fit (having congruence) with the methodology and aim of the study. Often there is overlap

BOX 4.4 ■ A Brief Overview of Some Key Qualitative Methodologies/Approaches

Grounded Theory

Grounded theory is an approach in which the researcher "derives a general, abstract theory of a process, action, or interaction grounded in the views of participants in a study" (Creswell and Creswell 2018, p. 248). Interviews, focus groups, and document review are commonly used methods, and data collection and data analysis occur simultaneously (Glasper and Rees 2017, p. 81) whereby the interaction between analysis, theory building, and subsequent data collection is central to developing a theory that is grounded in the data.

Narrative Inquiry

Narrative research is an approach or a family of approaches in which the "researcher studies the lives of individuals and asks one or more to provide stories about their lives" (Creswell and Creswell 2018, p. 249). The primary way of generating stories is through interviews; they can be single or longitudinal and aim to generate depth of context. The researcher's engagement with the storyteller inevitably shapes the story (Glasper and Rees, 2017, p. 109). The researcher retells or re-stories the information that has been shared.

Phenomenological Research

Phenomenological research is an approach in which the researcher "identifies the essence of human experiences about a phenomenon as described by the participants in a study" (Creswell and Creswell, 2018, p. 249). It is concerned with the "lifeworld" or lived experience of individuals (Glasper and Rees, 2017, p. 78) and gaining a deep understanding of the meaning or nature of meaning of everyday experiences.

Ethnographic Research

Ethnographic research is an approach in which the researcher "studies an intact cultural group in a natural setting over a prolonged period of time by collecting primarily observational and interview data" (Creswell and Creswell, 2018, p. 247). It aims to generate an understanding of attitudes, beliefs, and practices by uncovering "insider views" by the researcher watching, listening, and questioning what is observed (Glasper and Rees 2017, p. 75) and trying to make sense of how a group, community, or culture operates.

Case Study Research

Case study research is an approach in which the researcher "explores in depth a program, event, activity, process, or one or more individuals. The case(s) are bounded by time and activity, and researchers collect detailed information using a variety of data collections procedures over a sustained period of time" (Creswell and Creswell, 2018, p. 247). It is an in-depth investigation that aims to understand the "how" and "why" of the selected phenomenon. The boundaries of a case are defined by determining its parameters, such as the person(s), the geographical area, the specific event, the setting, organization, or incidence (Glasper and Rees, 2017, p. 84).

Participatory Research

Participatory research is an approach in which the researcher co-constructs knowledge and meaning with his or her participants, and it is based on the premise that the participants are "experts in their own lives." Participatory research uses methods that promote the active and engaged participation of people in generating knowledge and promoting change. Participatory research is often seen as the approach of choice for hard to reach or marginalized groups such as children and young people (Coyne and Carter, 2018).

Action Research

Action research is an approach in which the researcher adopts a range of methods and engages with stakeholders to undertake transformative research together in an "open-ended cycle of identifying a problem, imagining, then implementing a solution, evaluating the experience with a focus on both the problem and the solution, then changing practice(s) according to what has been learned" (Elliot et al., 2016). It aims to be empowering with the intention of improving the stakeholders' social situations.

Appreciative Inquiry

Appreciative inquiry is an approach in which the researcher uses an "affirmative, collaborative, relational and democratic approach to their research… it has some similarities to action research… [but it differs as it]… actively adopts an appreciative stance" (Glasper and Rees, 2017, p. 110). It is "founded on the simple assumption that human systems—teams, organizations and people—move in the direction of what they study, what they focus upon and what they talk about with regularity" (www.positivechange.org/how-we-work/appreciative-inquiry-ai/).

BOX 4.5 ■ **A Brief Overview of Four Key Categories of Qualitative Data-Collection Methods**

Verbal Research Methods

Verbal methods include interviews (ranging from in-depth/focused interviews to semi-structured interviews), narratives, focus groups, small-group discussions, activity-oriented approaches, and diaries.

Observational Research Methods

Observation can be undertaken with the researcher adopting different roles ranging from participant observation where the researcher engages in the situation or setting, to a more passive role where the researcher watches the behaviors and talk that occurs within the setting but does not become engaged.

Visual and Arts-Based Research Methods

Visual methods draw on approaches such as photography, drawing, film, video, and performance.

Documentary Materials

Documentary methods include newspapers, existing diaries, reports and records, media, and autobiographies.

---

between methods, for example, observation requires the researcher to observe what is happening and to note what is said. Visual methods that generate drawings or photographs are often linked with discussion and exploration of the images. The context in which an interview takes place requires the researcher to make note of the setting and surroundings. An examination of diaries and newspaper reports may be linked to exploration of similar stories on film. Where this overlap occurs, this should be made explicit.

A range of factors need to be considered in relation to the methods utilized (Table 4.2). The methods used should be consistent with the specific methodological framework within which the study was located. So, if a phenomenological study aims to explore, "What is this or that kind of experience like?" (van Manen, 1990, p. 9), the methods of data collection should reflect this aim; thus, if postal questionnaires were utilized that comprised mainly closed questions, you might question the depth of detail obtained and the credibility of the findings. Similar concerns might be raised if a researcher described conducting an observational study based on a single short episode of observation.

When appraising a paper, you need to look to see if there is a clear indication of why each method of data collection was chosen. If more than one technique was utilized (multiple methods), this should be justified. You should be able to identify how many phases of data collection took place: was it, for example, a series of single interviews that took place during one period, a series of interviews that took place at several time points, or interviews followed up with focus groups? The rationale for each data-collection phase (if there was more than one) should be clear, and there should be an explanation of why and when things took place and how the phases linked together.

ETHICS

Clearly, good qualitative research design is contingent on a good ethical and moral stance being adopted by the researcher (Carter, 2008, Morse, 2015) and diligent consideration of the risks to participants, settings, and the researcher. Ethical issues can occur throughout a study. Careful preparation of study design and study materials, adopting a reflexive perspective, identifying potential power relationships, and ensuring that participants are respected, are ways of ensuring ethical and moral integrity within a qualitative study.

Reflexivity, defined as the process of "critical self-reflection" that the researcher undertakes to consider his or her "biases, theoretical predispositions, preferences, and so forth" (Schwandt,

TABLE 4.2 ■ Factors to Consider in Relation to Methods

Question	Examples
What method(s) was used?	It should be clear whether data were collected via single or multiple methods. It is common in qualitative research for a number of different methods to be used in a single study. An observational study may include observation, interviews with key informants, and examination of documents and texts.
How was the method used?	The way in which methods are used will vary. Interviews and focus groups may be semi-structured and guided by a schedule or adopt a more open narrative approach in which a single question is posed to stimulate discussion. Observation may be conducted from the stance of a participant involved in the processes being observed, or as a non-participant in a less engaged way. The description of the chosen method should enable you to understand clearly what was done and how; it should be congruent with the aim of the study, the methodology, and the theoretical perspective.
Where did data collection take place?	A characteristic of qualitative research is that it is naturalistic. However, it is carried out in a range of settings that have the potential to influence the information obtained. For example, if a study exploring compliance with treatment took place in the clinical setting where treatment was provided, this may influence what participants felt able to say.
Who was involved in data collection, and if multiple people how was consistency assured?	An indication should be given of who was involved in data collection. For example, if a study not only took place in a clinical setting but also was conducted by the person responsible for providing the treatment, then even more concerns should be raised relating to the credibility of the findings. If several researchers were involved in collecting data, they may be collecting it in different ways or asking totally different questions. You might want to explore how a degree of consistency was maintained.
How long did data collection last, and was the duration of engagement commensurate with the aims of the study?	In returning to Lincoln and Guba's (1985) criteria for assessing the trustworthiness of a study, credibility is enhanced by prolonged engagement in the field. Phenomenological and ethnographic studies aim to elicit rich and deep insights. If interviews were conducted that only lasted 20 minutes or a single observation was undertaken, you might question the depth of insight obtained.

2015), is key within qualitative research due to its acceptance that knowledge is co-constructed between the researcher and the participants and that the researchers' values and biases are inevitably present. So, for example, a researcher's cultural background may position him or her within the group he or she is researching or outside of it.

One key element of positioning is that the researcher is often in a privileged position compared with the participant. This may occur if a researcher recruits participants from his or her own caseload, and therefore his or her relationship with participants may influence the information provided or the questions a researcher may have felt able to ask. Similarly, power imbalances may occur between an adult researcher and a child participant, or a senior manager and a more junior employee, or in any situation or setting in which the researcher may be perceived by the participant to be able to exert influence.

Any potential power imbalance is something that needs to be considered when appraising a study. Potential power imbalances and other such issues can be addressed by involving the public in the development, undertaking, and reporting of research (Glasper and Rees 2017, p. 28). This is separate to the recruitment of people to participate in the study itself.

Ensuring that the research participants' voices and ideas are represented in the research is key to ensuring that the participants are respected and heard and also to allowing the reader to appraise whether the researcher's interpretations authentically arise from the data. The voices of participants can be evident in quotations and other materials such as photographs, drawings, and film clips that appear in or are linked to in the paper/report.

SAMPLING AND RECRUITMENT

A sample may comprise, among other things, people, sites/settings, environments, organizations, documents, the Internet, or visual material. Sampling is the process by which a subset (e.g., of the target population) is selected (LoBiondo-Wood and Haber, 2018). In qualitative research, nonprobability sampling is used and the sample size is usually small (in terms of the number of individuals or sites selected) to ensure that the researcher can "collect extensive detail about the individuals or sites studied" (Creswell and Poth, 2018, p. 327). Conscious choices will have been made regarding the population from which the sample was drawn, the size, and relevant characteristics or features. In critically appraising a study, questions should focus on why and how these decisions were made, the impact that the sample had on the findings, and the implications in terms of the transferability of the findings to other contexts. A number of approaches to sampling are used, the most common of which are purposive, theoretical, convenience, and snowball sampling (Box 4.6).

The researcher should make it clear what decisions and choices informed the size of the sample; this will help you appraise how this may have affected the data generated. The transferability of the study can be assessed by the level of description given about the sample. To say that an

---

BOX 4.6 ■ A Brief Overview of Some Key Sampling Approaches

Purposive Sampling

Occurs when participants, settings, or documents are selected because they have specific characteristics or features that will enhance understanding of the research topic and because they are perceived to be typical of the population of interest (Lobiondo-Wood and Harper, 2018). These are identified before the commencement of the study and monitored as the recruitment progresses. You should be able to identify clearly the characteristics chosen and determine their relevance to the aim of the study and any impact they may have on its transferability.

Theoretical Sampling

Often associated with grounded theory as the sample evolves during data collection. An initial, often homogenous sample, will be selected and a period of data collection and analysis undertaken. A further heterogenous sample is then determined informed by the analysis of the first data set. This process continues until 'data saturation', the point at which nothing new is emerging (Lobiondo-Wood and Harper, 2018). In critiquing this approach, you need to see that data collection, analysis, and recruitment occurred as an iterative process and be convinced that data saturation was reached.

Convenience Sampling

Occurs when a researcher chooses a sample because it is easy to access, for example, the first people the researcher meets within a setting or those available on a particular day. It is important to look at the influence this will have on the data collected. Recruiting in this way is not necessarily wrong, but you should (i) be aware of the potential impact of this decision on the data generated and (ii) be reassured that the researcher has taken account of and tried to minimize any potential impact this may have had.

Snowball Sampling

Occurs when the researcher invites an existing participant to suggest another person or site who might be eligible to participate in the study and who would be "information rich" (Creswell and Poth, 2018, p. 159). Snowball sampling relies on the participant's existing knowledge and networks.

observational study was conducted "in a busy outpatient clinic" says little about the setting, or saying that "eight women took part in the study" explains nothing about the women. The researcher should enable you to understand who was involved in the generation of the data.

If a sample comprises people, the process of recruitment should be clear, enabling you to assess any impact this may have had on who declined or participated in the study.

DATA ANALYSIS

The way in which analysis is undertaken within qualitative studies can sit uncomfortably with people who are used to a more quantitative approach. Interpretation built on the researcher's iterative exploration of the data is fundamental to qualitative research. Rigorous qualitative work does not simply report or describe what the researcher has gained from their data, but it goes beyond this to a deeper conceptual engagement.

In terms of evidence of depth of analysis, you need to question if the analysis moves iteratively (back and forward) through a non-linear process during which data are organized and read, emergent ideas are recorded, codes are developed and classed into themes, interpretations are developed and assessed, and the data are represented and visualized to provide an account of the findings. This process has been called a "data analysis spiral" (Creswell and Poth, 2018, p. 185–186). This iterative approach aims to ensure that the findings have depth of meaning and that the research extends our understanding rather than simply being a superficial description. For example, a findings section may identify that five themes were created and may provide a description of each theme, illustrated with in-text quotes, but you may be left asking yourself "so what" because the author has not gone on to interpret their meaning.

Holloway and Galvin (2017) propose that researchers should provide evidence of an audit trail throughout the analysis to enable someone else to gain insight into the process and decisions that were made. Although comprehensive access to this audit trail will not be available to the appraiser, reference to this trail should be made in the paper. Different approaches to analysis can be adopted (Box 4.7).

BOX 4.7 ■ A Brief Overview of Analytical Approaches

Thematic Analysis

"Is a generic approach to data analysis … that allows researchers theoretical flexibility …[and] refers to a search for patterns in a data set and is particularly based in language and meaning" (Holloway and Galvin, 2017, p. 294). It draws codes into groups, the groups into sub-themes, the sub-themes into themes, and then the themes into a global theme that pulls everything together.

Grounded Theory Analysis

Is an inductive approach to analysis in which data collection, analysis, and theory development are inter-related. The analysis process encompasses open, axial, and selective coding that is undertaken to inform the development of a substantive theory (Creswell and Poth, 2018).

Framework Analysis

Is "an analytical method closely related to thematic analysis but involving highly structured coding of qualitative data in matrices of codes. The framework method involves first planning a study and gathering data, second arranging topics of analysis into an analytical framework, third coding the data according to that framework, and then systematically charting the data into the data matrix" (Elliot et al., 2016). This process aims to inform the development of descriptive and explanatory account.

Narrative Analysis

Is the "analysis of the stories people tell to themselves and each other… [i]t pays particular attention to the way narratives are structured according to cultural rules, local conventions, and the influence of other narratives" (Elliot et al., 2016). It focuses on the identification meaning of stories.

BOX 4.8 ■ A Brief Overview of Approaches to Trustworthiness in Data Analysis

Member Checking (Participant Validation)

Provides the opportunity for the people involved in the generation of the data to review it and to explore their agreement (or not) with the way in which they are being represented; Birt et al. (2016) propose that synthesized member checking addresses some of the issues that arise as a result of the tendency to use member checking. Member checking can happen in a number of different ways, but typically this involves returning the transcript or a summary of an interview to the participant for comment or asking for comments on the draft of a report.

Search for Negative Cases

Searching for negative cases is a means of increasing the credibility of analysis and the trustworthiness of the findings. This requires a researcher to explore and report on situations, experiences, or points of view "that do not easily fit into the developing theory or their own ideas"; thus forcing the researcher to rethink their ideas and consider alternative explanations, ensuring that the final findings are as "valid and plausible" as they can be (Holloway and Galvin, 2017, p. 313).

Triangulation

Is the "process by which the phenomenon of topic under study is examined from different perspectives...findings of one type of method (or data, researcher, theory) can be checked out by reference to another" (Holloway and Galvin, 2017, p. 314).

There are a number of steps that can be undertaken to increase the trustworthiness of the analysis. These include member checking, searching for negative cases, peer review (peer debriefing), triangulation, audit/decision trail, thick description, prolonged engagement, and reflexivity. Some of these are presented in Box 4.8. However, as noted earlier, some of these markers of trustworthiness are contested (Denzin, 2018) and some authors warn of the unintended consequences for the research, especially if they are used uncritically and non-reflexively (Varpio et al., 2016).

FINDINGS, CONCLUSIONS, CONTRIBUTION, AND REPORTING THE STUDY

The findings and conclusions of the study are key elements to appraise, as these are core to the contribution to knowledge claimed by the authors. These all need to be considered in the context of the aim of the study, theoretical/interpretive perspective, methodology, and approach to analysis. The findings of the study need to be presented in such a way that it is clear that they arise out of the data analysis and are presented with sufficient context to provide a clear and rich description.

If using trustworthiness criteria as a guide to demonstrating the quality of their research, the researchers need to provide evidence of the credibility, transferability, dependability, and confirmability of their research (see Table 4.1).

Conclusion

Good qualitative research is thorough, reliable, rigorous, explanatory, transparent, reflexive, and, according to Brown (2010), undertaken by informed and confident researchers. We have provided an overview of the core knowledge domains for the appraisal of qualitative studies; these domains are evident to a greater or lesser extent in standardized checklists. Reading qualitative research will require you to consider the choices and decisions made by the researcher, the consistency between all elements of the study, and the fit with the findings. Appraising qualitative research requires the appraiser to be open to the interpretations presented by the researcher while maintaining a critical stance.

Exercise

We encourage you to consolidate your learning by undertaking the exercise on the website.

References

Audrey, S., 2011. Qualitative research in evidence-based medicine: improving decision-making and participation in randomized controlled trials of cancer treatments. Palliat. Med. 25 (8), 758–765.

Birt, L., Scott, S., Cavers, D., Campbell, C., Walter, F., 2016. Member checking: a tool to enhance trustworthiness or merely a nod to validation? Qual. Health Res. 26 (13), 1802–1811.

Blaikie, N., 2009. Designing social research, second ed. Polity Press, Cambridge.

Brown, A.P., 2010. Qualitative method and compromise in applied social research. Qual. Res. 10 (2), 229–248.

Carter, B., 2008. "Good" and "bad" stories: decisive moments, "shock and awe" and being moral. J. Clin. Nurs. 17 (8), 1063–1070.

Chenail, R.J., 2011. Learning to appraise the quality of qualitative research articles: a contextualised learning object for constructing knowledge. Qual. Rep. 16 (1), 236–248.

Coffey, L., Mooney, O., Dunne, S., et al., 2016. Cancer survivors' perspectives on adjustment-focused self-management interventions: a qualitative meta-synthesis. J. Cancer Surviv. 10 (6), 1012–1034.

Cohen, D., Crabtree, B., 2006. Using qualitative methods in healthcare research. A comprehensive guide for designing, writing, reviewing and reporting qualitative research. Qualitative Research Guidelines Project. Robert Wood Johnson Foundation, Princeton, NJ. Available from: http://www.qualres.org/. Accessed 20.08.18.

Cooper, C., O'Cathain, A., Hind, D., Adamson, J., Lawton, J., Baird, W., 2014. Conducting qualitative research within Clinical Trials Units: avoiding potential pitfalls. Contemp. Clin. Trials 38 (2), 338–343.

Coyne, I., Carter, B., 2018. Being Participatory. Researching with Children and Young People. Springer, Switzerland.

Creswell, J.W., Creswell, J.D., 2018. Research Design: Qualitative, Quantitative, and Mixed Methods approaches, fifth ed. Sage Publications, Thousand Oaks, CA.

Creswell, J.W., Poth, C.N., 2018. Qualitative Inquiry and Research Design. Choosing Among Five Approaches, fourth ed. Sage Publications, Thousand Oaks, CA.

Critical Appraisal Skills Programme, 2018. CASP Qualitative Checklist. Available from: https://casp-uk.net/casp-tools-checklists/. Accessed 12.11.2018.

Denzin, N.K., 2018. The elephant in the living room, or extending the conversation about the politics of evidence. In: Denzin, N.K., Lincoln, Y.S. (Eds.), The SAGE Handbook of Qualitative Research, fifth ed. Sage Publications, Thousand Oaks, CA, p. 968.

Elliot, M., Fairweather, I., Olsen, W., Pampaka, M., 2016. A Dictionary of Social Research Methods. Oxford University Press, Oxford.

Farquhar, M.C., Ewing, G., Booth, S., 2011. Using mixed methods to develop and evaluate complex interventions in palliative care research. Palliat. Med. 25 (8), 748–757.

Glasper, E.A., Rees, C. (Eds.), 2017. Nursing and Healthcare Research at a Glance. Wiley-Blackwell, Oxford.

Griffin, G., 2017. A Dictionary of Gender Studies. Oxford University Press, Oxford.

Hannes, K., Lockwood, C., Pearson, A., 2010. A comparative analysis of three online appraisal instruments' ability to assess validity in qualitative research. Qual. Health Res. 20 (12), 1736–1743.

Holloway, I., Galvin, K., 2017. Qualitative research in nursing and healthcare, fourth ed. Blackwell Publishing Ltd, Oxford.

Kornhaber, R., de Jong, A.E.E., McLean, L., 2015. Rigorous, robust and systematic: qualitative research and its contribution to burn care. An integrative review. Burns 41 (8), 1619–1626.

Kozleski, E.B., 2017. The uses of qualitative research: powerful methods to inform evidence-based practice in education. Res. Pract. Persons Severe Disabl. 42 (1), 14.

La Caze, A., 2016. The hierarchy of evidence and quantum theory. J. Clin. Epidemiol. 72, 4–6.

Lau, S.R., Traulsen, J.M., 2017. Are we ready to accept the challenge? Addressing the shortcomings of contemporary qualitative health research. Res. Social. Adm. Pharm. 13 (2), 332–338.

Lewin, S., Booth, A., Glenton, C., et al., 2018a. Applying GRADE-CERQual to qualitative evidence synthesis findings: introduction to the series. Implement. Sci. 13 (Suppl 1), 2.

Lewin, S., Bohren, M., Rashidian, A., et al., 2018b. Applying GRADE-CERQual to qualitative evidence synthesis findings-paper 2: how to make an overall CERQual assessment of confidence and create a Summary of Qualitative Findings table. Implement. Sci. 13 (Suppl 1), 10.

Lincoln, Y.S., Guba, E.G., 1985. Naturalistic Inquiry. Sage Publications, Newbury Park.

Lobiondo-Wood, G., Haber, J., 2018. Nursing Research. Methods and Critical Appraisal for Evidence-Based Practice, ninth ed. Elsevier, St. Louis.

Morse, J., 2015. Critical analysis of strategies for determining rigor in qualitative inquiry. Qual. Health Res. 25 (9), 11.

Pearson, A., 2010. Evidence-based healthcare and qualitative research. J. Res. Nurs. 15 (6), 489–493.

Porter, S., 2010. The role of qualitative research in evidence-based policy and practice. J.Res.Nurs. 15 (6), 495–496.

Porter, S., Millar, C., Reid, J., 2012. Cancer cachexia care: the contribution of qualitative research to evidence-based practice. Cancer Nurs. 35 (6), E30–E38.

Ravitch, S.M., Mittenfelner, N.C., 2016. Qualitative Research: Bridging the Conceptual, Theoretical, and Methodological. Sage Publications, Los Angeles.

Richter-Montpetit, M., 2018. Queer theory. In: Brown, G., McLean, I., McMillan, A. (Eds.), Concise Oxford Dictionary of Politics and International Relations, fourth ed. Oxford University Press, Oxford.

Roller, M.R., Lavrakas, P.L., 2015. Applied Qualitative Research Design. A Total Quality Framework Approach. The Guilford Press, New York.

Santiago-Delefosse, M., Gavin, A., Bruchez, C., Roux, P., Stephen, S.L., 2016. Quality of qualitative research in the health sciences: analysis of the common criteria present in 58 assessment guidelines by expert users. Soc. Sci. Med. 148, 142–151.

Schwandt, T.A., 2015. The SAGE dictionary of qualitative inquiry, fourth ed. Sage Publications, Los Angeles.

Stake, R.E., 2010. Qualitative Research. Studying How Things Work. Guilford Press, New York.

The Joanna Briggs Institute, 2017. Critical Appraisal Checklist for Qualitative Research. Available from: http://joannabriggs.org/research/critical-appraisal-tools.html. Accessed 12.11.2018.

Toews, I., Booth, A., Berg, R.C., et al., 2017. Further exploration of dissemination bias in qualitative research required to facilitate assessment within qualitative evidence syntheses. J. Clin. Epidemiol. 88, 133–139.

Toles, M., Barroso, J., 2018. Introduction to Qualitative Research. In: Lobiondo-Wood, G., Haber, J. (Eds.), Nursing Research. Methods and Critical Appraisal for Evidence-Based Practice, ninth ed. Elsevier, St Louis, pp. 88–101.

Tong, A., Flemming, K., McInnes, E., Oliver, S., Craig, J., 2012. Enhancing transparency in reporting the synthesis of qualitative research: ENTREQ. BMC Med. Res. Methodol. 12, 181.

Tong, A., Sainsbury, P., Craig, J., 2007. Consolidated criteria for reporting qualitative research (COREQ): a 32-item checklist for interviews and focus groups. Int. J. Qual. Health Care 19 (6), 349–357.

Tracy, S.J., 2010. Qualitative quality: eight "big-tent" criteria for excellent qualitative research. Qual. Inq. 16 (10), 837–851.

van Manen, M., 1990. Researching lived experience, human science for an action sensitive pedagogy. State University of New York Press, New York.

van Wijngaarden, E., Meide, H.V., Dahlberg, K., 2017. Researching health are as a meaningful practice: toward a nondualistic view on evidence for qualitative research. Qual. Health Res. 27 (11), 1738–1747.

Varpio, L., Ajjawi, R., Monrouxe, L.V., O'Brien, B.C., Rees, C.E., 2017. Shedding the cobra effect: problematising thematic emergence, triangulation, saturation and member checking. Med. Educ. 51 (1), 40–50.

Webster, F., Christian, J., Mansfield, E., et al., 2015. Capturing the experiences of patients across multiple complex interventions: a meta-qualitative approach. BMJ Open 5 (9), e007664.

CHAPTER 5

Using Evidence from Quantitative Studies

Gillian A. Lancaster ■ Gareth McCray

KEY POINTS

- Quantitative research involves the collection and analysis of numerical information.
- It can be useful to consider the "hierarchy of evidence" when identifying the most appropriate (quantitative) research design for your clinical practice question.
- Understanding how to critically appraise research studies is a core skill for those wanting to use research evidence to inform their practice.
- Critical appraisal entails assessing the quality of a study, interpreting the results, and deciding on the applicability of the results to your setting or patient group.
- There are various checklists to help with critical appraisal, and they are specific to the type of study design.
- In this chapter, we use critical appraisal checklists to assess the quality of studies that ask questions about (i) the effectiveness of a therapy or intervention, (ii) the performance of a diagnostic test or method of assessment, and (iii) the likely prognosis of a particular health problem or disease in relation to a defined set of risk factors.
- Developing a clinically useful interpretation of study results is important:
    - Results from a study about the effectiveness of therapies may be reported as odds ratios, risk ratios, relative risk reductions, absolute risk reductions, and the number needed to treat.
    - Results from a study about the accuracy of a diagnostic test or assessment may be reported as sensitivity, specificity, likelihood ratios, and pre- and post-test odds.
    - Results from a study about prognosis or harm may be reported as the number needed to harm.
    - Confidence intervals as well as "p-values" are commonly reported.
- Understanding how these results are calculated and/or interpreted will allow you to judge whether the conclusions that the author has drawn are indeed supported by the study findings.
- A key step in critical appraisal is deciding whether the results of a study are applicable to your patients and clinical setting.

Introduction

Quantitative research is a methodology based on experimentation and observation in which numerical information is collected, using, for example, questionnaires or structured interviews, or is extracted from existing databases such as disease registries or other large surveys. Different research questions require evaluation through different study designs. Randomized controlled trials (RCTs) are the "gold standard" study design for primary research on which to base decisions on the effectiveness of healthcare interventions, but they are not appropriate, or ethical, for answering all clinical questions. Observational study designs such as cohort studies, case-control studies, and cross-sectional surveys define the nature of inquiry when we want to observe what is going on in the population of interest but we are not going to intervene in any way. A cohort study, for example, may be conducted prospectively and longitudinally, following and recording the progress of a cohort of participants over a number of years to see whether, in the light of their exposure history, they become diseased. This enables prediction of the likely prognosis or health outcome given a certain set of risk factors. On the other hand, for a case-control study, we retrospectively go back in time to gather information on groups of diseased participants (cases) and non-diseased participants (controls) to compare whether or not having been exposed to certain risk factors for disease earlier in life (e.g., smoking history, exposure to sunburn as a child) has a bearing on getting the disease. Cross-sectional surveys observe a cross-section of people at some point or period in time to gain a "snapshot" of what is going on in the population in terms of the prevalence of certain diseases, for example. Each design, therefore, has a slightly different strategy behind it.

There is no such thing as a perfect research study. Research is a real-world process, and this means that researchers are often forced to compromise on certain aspects of the research and to modify the study design for lots of legitimate reasons. Similarly, it is important to realize that research is done on samples of a population who will never be identical to patients attending a community clinic or the patients in a ward. When designing a research study, researchers have to consider a number of key questions (Box 5.1). These questions apply in every type of research design. The decisions made by the researchers in response to these questions directly affect the degree to which the results of a study may be affected by bias. Bias refers to any influence or action in a study that distorts the findings (Gray et al., 2016). In other words, it is any factor—for example, the way the sample is collected (selection bias) or the past length of time over which people are being asked to remember certain information (recall bias)—that leads to interventions appearing to be effective or risk factors for disease harmless when in fact they are not, or vice versa. The critical reader of research must always be aware that there may be multiple explanations for the findings reported in a study (O'Mathuna, 2014). Strategies for the minimization of bias are now well known, and different strategies are required for different research designs and for the different stages of the study (Malone et al., 2014).

Hierarchy of Evidence

Evidence that some research designs are more powerful than others has given rise to the notion of a hierarchy of evidence (Summerskill, 2001). Fig. 5.1 illustrates this hierarchy for studies relating to experimental designs that assess the effectiveness of therapies or interventions and for observa-

---

BOX 5.1 ■ Questions to Be Considered in the Design of a Research Study

What information (entities and variables) should be examined?
Under what conditions should this information be examined and collected?
What type(s) of data should be collected?
From whom should we collect these data?
At what time points (including follow-up) should data be collected?
What method should be employed for data collection?
How will the data be analyzed?

Modified from Sim, J., Wright, C., 2000. Basic elements of research design. In: Sim, J., Wright, C. (Ed.). Research in Health-Care: Concepts, Designs and Methods. Nelson Thornes: Cheltenham.

tional study designs that study known risk factors for disease. The higher a methodology appears on the continuum in the hierarchy, the more likely the results of such methods are to represent objective reality and hence the more certainty the practitioner has that the effect of interest will produce the associated health outcome (O'Mathuna, 2014). Such hierarchies provide a useful "rule of thumb" against which to grade studies. The Oxford Centre for Evidence-Based Medicine is a good resource for more detailed information on levels of evidence (see https://www.cebm.net /2016/05/ocebm-levels-of-evidence/).

When looking for evidence about the effectiveness of interventions, well-conducted systematic reviews of RCTs or well-conducted RCTs provide the highest form of evidence. The process of randomization means that the observed differences between the intervention group and the comparison group are more likely to be due to the intervention and not to other factors, such as patient, nurse, or doctor preference (Matthews, 2006). There will, however, always be circumstances in which randomization may be inappropriate or impossible, particularly in health service research (Bowling, 2014). An obvious example is studies about harm or prognosis in which it would not be ethical to give subjects a substance that was thought to be hazardous to their health.

The hierarchy of evidence shown in Fig. 5.1 has, in the past, led some clinicians to expressing concerns that the only questions considered to be important are those about effectiveness of interventions, and that the only valid type of study is the RCT (Evans and Pearson, 2001; French 2002). In circumstances in which there are clear reasons for not randomizing, as we have seen already, observational studies have a vital role in providing evidence (Faraoni and Schaefer, 2016). Furthermore, it would be inappropriate to conduct an RCT to answer a question such as "How do young people with cancer experience and manage fatigue?" Here the study aims to examine the experience of fatigue and explore influencing factors and management strategies adopted by young people with cancer, so a qualitative approach may be more appropriate.

In Fig. 5.1, systematic reviews of RCTs feature at the top of the hierarchy of evidence about the effectiveness of interventions. Systematic reviews are discussed in depth in Chapter 7, so it suffices to simply clarify at this point that a systematic review uses explicit and rigorous methods

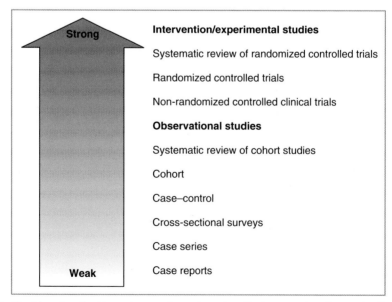

Fig. 5.1 The hierarchy of evidence for questions about the effectiveness of an intervention/therapy or observed risk factors for disease.

to identify, assess, and synthesize pertinent research evidence on a defined health question. This is in contrast to a traditional literature review, which might simply reflect the findings of a few papers that support an author's particular point of view. For the busy practitioner, the most important advantage to systematic reviews would seem to be their potential for aiding translation of research evidence into practice, through informing clinical practice guidelines, action sets, and care policies (see Chapter 8). A well-conducted review can help overcome many of the limitations of individual studies (Egger et al., 2001).

Why Is Critical Appraisal Necessary?

On a daily basis, nurses and other healthcare professionals are faced with a range of important clinical decisions. Practice based on evidence can decrease the uncertainty that patients and healthcare professionals experience in a complex and constantly evolving healthcare system. Not all published research evidence can be used for making decisions about patient care. Deficiencies in research design can make an intervention look better than it really is (Matthews, 2006). In addition, the location and participants of a particular research study may affect the results in a unique way. It is therefore necessary to assess the quality, interpretation of results, and applicability of any research evidence that is being consulted to answer a specific clinical question. The process used to do this is known as *critical appraisal* and is a core skill for those wanting to use evidence in their practice.

As discussed in Chapter 1, clinical decisions are influenced not only by research evidence, but also by clinical expertise and patient preference. A variety of appraisal approaches can be used to determine the certainty and applicability of knowledge underpinning each of these three aspects of decision-making (Stevens, 2014). In this chapter, we focus on the appraisal of research evidence only and, specifically, quantitative research evidence. So, how do you critically appraise evidence produced through quantitative research designs? What does it demand of you?

Critical appraisal can be broken down into three distinct but related parts, as illustrated in Fig. 5.2.

1. Are the results of the study valid? In other words, is the quality of the study good enough to produce results that can be used to inform clinical decisions?
2. What are the results, and what do they mean for my patients?
3. Can I apply the results locally in my clinical setting?

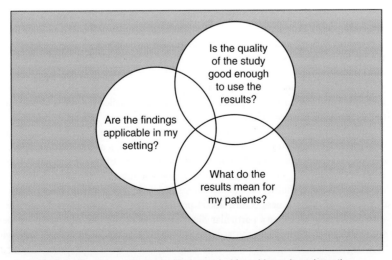

Fig. 5.2 The three aspects of critical appraisal for evidence-based practice.

Answering "yes" or "no" to these questions can prove a challenge to healthcare practitioners. This observation by Oxman et al., made in 1993, remains equally pertinent today: research evidence comes in shades of gray, rather than black and white: results *may* be valid, *might* show clinically important findings, *perhaps* will improve the patient's outcome.

Over the past 25 years or so, researchers and clinicians around the world have been working together to develop standard approaches to addressing these three questions. This work has led to the development of quality criteria for assessing the design of research studies. These criteria have been incorporated into critical appraisal checklists in the form of streamlined guides and toolkits that make the process of assessing studies much easier. See for example the Critical Appraisal Skills Programme website (https://casp-uk.net/) and the "Resources" section of the Centre for Evidence Based Medicine website (www.cebm.net).

This chapter provides help in developing the skills and knowledge necessary to critically appraise quantitative studies and uses practical examples and exercises to illustrate the process (see website).

Are the Results of the Study Valid/Is the Quality of the Study Good Enough to Produce Results that can be Used?

One of the issues that all researchers face in the design and conduct of research in real-world settings is that of choosing a study design to minimize bias. Strategies adopted by the researchers to minimize bias should be evident in the reporting of the research. Critical appraisal checklists are designed to summarize the bias minimization strategies and help practitioners to ask the most relevant questions that will lead to a decision about the quality and usefulness of a paper.

As shown in Chapter 2, the process of critical appraisal for evidence-based practice starts with the formulation of a question that arises from clinical practice. For critical appraisal purposes, clinical practice questions can, broadly speaking, be categorized into different types. In this chapter, we focus on clinical questions about the following:

- The effectiveness of a therapy or intervention
- The accuracy of a diagnostic test or other method of assessment
- The prognosis of a particular disease or health problem in relation to a given set of associated risk factors

For each type of question, there is a corresponding "most appropriate" research design (overall plan or structure used by the researcher) that can be used to answer the question with a known degree of precision and minimal risk of bias (Blaikie 2009).

In this chapter we have focused on the optimal study design for three different types of questions, as illustrated in Table 5.1. However, it is important to remember that there may be good reasons why researchers choose to use study designs that at first appear to be less appropriate for the research question. Each research project presents unique challenges and a certain degree of flexibility is required by the researcher.

If the clinical question is about whether a particular intervention (e.g., a nurse-led discharge package) produces a certain outcome (e.g., decreased hospital stay), a study that compares length of hospital stay in a group receiving the intervention with length of stay in a group not receiving the intervention is required. There are a number of possible research designs that could be used for such a study but large, multicenter RCTs (or a systematic review of RCTs) are likely to give the best evidence of effectiveness (Gray, 2009) provided they are conducted rigorously. In the case of questions about whether a particular diagnostic test or method of assessment performs well, a study design that compares the accuracy of a new test when used on people with and without the target condition against a reference standard will be most appropriate (Mant, 2004a).

TABLE 5.1 ■ **Matching Study Design to Question**

Type of Question	Example Question	Research Design
The effectiveness of a therapy or intervention	Does the use of electronic patient sensors in acutely ill adults admitted to intensive care optimize turning practices to reduce pressure injuries in these patients?	Randomized controlled trial
The performance or accuracy of a particular diagnostic test/method of assessment	In primary care, does asking pregnant women about feeling depressed, experiencing loss of interest and needing help accurately identify those who are clinically depressed?	Study investigating test accuracy in which a new method of assessment is compared with a reference standard test
Finding out the likely outcome of a particular health problem or disease in relation to a set of known risk factors (e.g., prognosis)	Are young adults recreationally using e-cigarettes at greater risk of initiating traditional cigarette smoking of tobacco?	Cohort study: participants exposed to an agent (electronic cigarette) are followed forward in time to see if they become traditional cigarette smokers. Case-control study: participants who are cigarette smokers are matched with controls (nonsmokers). Study looks back in time to identify exposure to an agent (electronic cigarette).

We will refer to this design as a diagnostic test study. Where the question is about the most likely outcome of a particular health problem (i.e., the prognosis) in the light of a number of associated risk factors, the most appropriate design will be one that measures relevant outcomes in individuals with (exposed to) and without (not exposed to) the relevant risk factor over a sufficient period of time (Mant 2004b). As we have already seen the appropriate study design for this type of question is the cohort study. In our exercises we will be using a set of checklists developed by the Critical Appraisal Skills Programme (https://casp-uk.net/casp-tools-checklists/) that have been created specifically to appraise these three different types of study design: namely (i) a randomized controlled trial (CASP 2018a), (ii) a diagnostic test study (CASP 2018b), and (iii) a cohort study (CASP 2018c).

Regardless of the type of study, a rigorous approach to the design, conduct, analysis and reporting stages of the study is important in view of the effect that each of these stages can have on the results. For example, RCTs with methodological shortfalls, such as failure to conceal from the patient and assessor the group to which the patient has been allocated, tend to overestimate treatment effects (Matthews 2006). Similarly diagnostic test studies that only choose a sample of confirmed diseased and non-diseased people and exclude the broad spectrum of people in between (e.g., with early mild or moderate symptoms), tend to inflate estimates of test performance (Lijmer et al., 1999).

General points to consider when assessing quality criteria for the three types of clinical question that we are considering are given in the following sections. These points should be considered when following the three examples in this chapter and when attempting the two exercises found on the website.

Points to Consider When Assessing the Quality of a Study that Asks a Question About the Effectiveness of a Therapy or Intervention

- The importance of randomization has already been discussed: it is a powerful technique in which the aim is to ensure that, as far as possible, the two groups are similar in every respect apart from the fact that one group is given the intervention and the other is not. This then means that any difference in outcome between the two groups is likely to be due to the intervention. A computer-generated random number sequence is one example of an appropriate randomization method. An approach that allocates people to the two groups (e.g., by treating on alternate days) is a weaker method of allocation, but may sometimes be the only feasible method.

- The group to which the patient has been allocated must be concealed from the clinician/researcher until the patient has (at least) been accepted into the trial. This is referred to as *allocation concealment* and is an important factor in reducing bias. If the clinician believes that the patient may benefit from the treatment and realizes that the patient is due to be allocated to the control group, he or she may consciously or subconsciously dissuade the patient from participating in the trial. Ideally, randomization should be carried out by someone independent of the project who may prepare, for example, sequentially numbered sealed, opaque envelopes containing the next treatment allocation. Clinical Trials Units (CTUs) can also provide this service. Allocation based on criteria such as date of birth or alternate days are not recommended as clinicians will be able to work out the next allocation sequence.

- Where possible, patients, clinicians, and researchers should continue to be "blinded" as to whether a patient is in the treatment or control group. If patients know that they are in the control group, they may feel that they have received substandard care and, as a result, may alter their behavior. Similarly, clinicians may consciously or subconsciously take compensatory measures for patients who are in the control group (for example, by offering alternative therapies or additional support). Any difference in the treatment effects between the two groups may be due to this additional attention rather than the intervention. A researcher may have preconceived ideas about the treatment and, where the outcomes of interest are fairly subjective, these preconceptions may influence the way in which the researcher analyzes and interprets the data. Clearly, blinding is not possible in all studies, but attempts should be made to blind one (single-blind) or all (double-blind/treble-blind) of the above groups of people.

- People drop out of studies for all sorts of reasons: death, move away from the area, treatment too unpleasant, and so on. It is important that the researcher tries to identify whether or not the reasons relate to the outcomes of interest, as this may have a bearing on the analysis. The analysis should ideally be done on an "intention-to-treat" basis: patients are analyzed in the groups to which they were randomized regardless of whether they swap from the intervention arm of the trial to the control arm or vice versa. If participants in the treatment group stop taking a drug because they feel worse (and blame the drug) and are then included in the control group, the drug may appear to be more effective than it really is due to exclusion of those patients with poor outcomes from the treatment group.

- Sample size is another important consideration. Did the researchers explicitly estimate how many people were needed to detect the minimum clinically worthwhile difference that they want to detect between groups? Studying more people than is necessary wastes resources, and studying too few people might lead to results that reflect chance variation rather than the real situation. To illustrate, in a trial of 10 participants, where five are randomized to receive drug A and five to receive drug B, and where the outcomes are the same for both groups, this could mean one of two things: either there is no difference between the drugs, or one of the drugs is more effective, but because of the small sample this difference is not detected (Kirkwood and Sterne, 2003). A "power calculation" will provide an estimate of the required sample size. The power of a study is the probability of detecting a significant result if the difference between outcomes in the two groups really exists.

- A descriptive summary of demographic and health status details for the two randomized groups is good practice at the start of the study. Apparent differences between the two groups, for example, differences in age, co-morbid conditions, gender, or disease severity, could potentially affect the results of the study. The groups should ideally be similar for any variables that are likely to influence outcome. Similarity between groups is not always achieved by randomization, even when the methods of randomization are adequate.

- It is helpful if the intervention is described in sufficient detail to allow clinicians to reproduce it in their own setting. In addition, the primary outcome in which the investigators would expect to see a clinically important difference should be given, along with details of how the outcome is to be measured. Measurement instruments that have been validated outside the study and found to measure what they purport to measure, and that are sensitive, appropriate, and acceptable, inspire more confidence than measurement instruments that have not been validated. Similarly, they should be consistently reliable when used on different occasions or by different assessors.

Points to Consider When Assessing the Quality of a Study that Asks a Question About the Performance or Accuracy of a Particular Diagnostic Test

- The "new" test should be compared against the method that is currently regarded as "the best" (i.e., the reference standard), and it is important that *both* tests are applied to all participants. It is also important that the reference standard correctly diagnoses participants because the "new" test is being compared in terms of its accuracy to this "gold standard."

- An appropriate spectrum of patients (i.e., patients with mild, moderate, and severe forms of the condition) should ideally be included in the study, with details of the proportions in each of these groups reported. A test may be able to identify people who are severely ill, but not those with a mild form of the condition.

- Ideally, a consecutive sample of participants who fulfill the inclusion criteria should be tested, or alternatively a random sample selected from a registry if such a list of participants is available. This ensures that individuals are not inappropriately "selected out" of the study, thereby affecting the results and conclusions of the study. The participants should be representative of the type of participants to which the test will be administered in practice and should be taken from the appropriate setting.

- It is recommended that the clinician or investigator is "blinded" to the results of the test that is carried out first. If the clinician suspects from the initial test that the patient does not have the disease in question, he or she may decide to avoid subjecting the patient to the second test. Blinding also avoids the conscious and unconscious bias of causing the reference standard to be overinterpreted when the diagnostic test is positive and underinterpreted when it is negative (Straus et al., 2019).

- Reliability (reproducibility) of a test needs to be considered: the results of tests carried out by different assessors or by the same assessor at different times should remain unchanged, provided the true underlying condition being measured (e.g., temperature) remains the same. Disagreement between two assessors is called *interobserver variability*, and disagreement within one assessor over time is called *intraobserver variability*. In tests that are not reproducible, it is difficult to know if a true measurement is being obtained. This creates problems in research and in clinical practice.

Points to Consider When Assessing the Quality of a Study that Asks a Question About the Likely Prognosis or Outcome of a Particular Health Problem or Disease in Relation to a Set of Risk Factors

- It is important that the participants in the study are truly "at risk" of getting the disease, and that they are entering the study disease-free, or at least at a common point in the course of their disease. In a cohort study aiming to identify the risk of renal disease in people with diabetes, for example, if some of the participants already have undiagnosed mild kidney damage at the start of the study, this could influence the results in a negative way. Entry or eligibility criteria are therefore required and should be clearly specified.
- Length of observation (or follow-up) should be adequate for all possible outcomes (especially negative outcomes). If participants, for example, people who have smoked 20 or more cigarettes a day for 1 year, are followed up for 4 years to establish risk of lung cancer, the conclusions of the study are likely to be very different than if followed up for 15 years.
- People are inevitably lost to follow-up during the course of a cohort study, and the reasons for this should be explored and closely monitored. If participants are lost to follow-up through death rather than because they feel better, and this information is known to the researcher, he or she can take this into consideration when presenting the results.
- Measurement of outcomes and exposures can be a source of bias, especially when the measure is subjective (e.g., quality of life) or sensitive (e.g., sexual abuse in childhood), or when a number of different assessors have taken measurements over the course of the study. The method of measurement should therefore be clearly defined in advance and regular training given as necessary. In addition, when measurement requires a degree of judgment, the person taking the measurement or doing the assessment should remain blind to the patient's condition.
- When observing health outcomes, it is important to take account of the factors or variables that can affect health. In longitudinal studies, time itself acts as a confounding variable. As people get older, they develop more illness regardless of any other factors. The effect of such confounding variables can be taken into account in the process of data analysis.

For a more detailed discussion of each set of points, readers are referred to the *Users' Guides to the Medical Literature* manual of the American Medical Association (Guyatt et al., 2015) or its more concise companion book (Guyatt et al., 2014).

To illustrate assessment of the quality of a research study, we use the clinical scenario given in Box 5.2, which is concerned with whether pressure injuries in acutely ill adults can be reduced by patients wearing a sensor to optimize turning practices. A search for evidence on the topic has revealed a paper by Pickham et al (2018). Table 5.2 shows our appraisal of the paper using criteria to assess the quality of the study that is asking a question about the effectiveness of an intervention.

What Do the Results of the Study Mean for My Patients?

Once you have decided the quality of the study is good enough to produce results that can be used to inform clinical decisions, the next stage is to interpret what the results of the study mean for your individual patients. This is the second aspect of critical appraisal (see Fig. 5.2). It is a common misperception that evidence-based practice is all about statistics. We hope that it is already clear that this is not the case. The evidence-based practice approach is that the statistical analyses carried out in a study are not the most important consideration when critically appraising a paper. Most important is the choice and quality of the study design. If a study was well designed for the research question being asked, then there is a high probability that the researchers' interpretation of the results can be trusted (Straus et al., 2019). Even well-conducted statistical analysis can-

---

BOX 5.2 ■ Example of a Study Assessing the Effectiveness of an Intervention

Scenario

Helen White is worried about her elderly mother, who has been admitted to intensive care after treatment for breast cancer. She doesn't want her mother to get pressure sores again like she did on a previous occasion in hospital. The nurse on the ward tells her that her mother could wear an electronic sensor to aid the nursing staff to remember to reposition her regularly while on the ward. She thinks this may be troublesome for her mother to wear and asks for your help in deciding what to do. You search for information on the web and find a relevant paper in the International Journal of Nursing.

Clinical Question

Do wearable patient sensors to promote optimal turning practices prevent pressure injuries in acutely ill adults admitted to intensive care?

Evidence

Pickham, D., Berte, N., Pihulic, A., Valdez, A., Mayer, B., 2018. Effect of a wearable patient sensor on care delivery for preventing pressure injuries in acutely ill adults: a pragmatic randomized clinical trial (LS-HAPI study). Int. J. Nurs. Stud. 80, 12–19.

Results Reported in the Study

The results for hospital-acquired pressure injuries (HAPI) are presented. For those patients allocated to wear the sensor in treatment mode (intervention group), 5 of 659 (0.7%) had one or more HAPIs compared with 15 of 653 (2.3%) patients wearing the sensor in control mode (control group).

---

not compensate for bias caused by deficiencies in the study design. When critically appraising a research study, the reader does not have to be an expert in statistics. However, it is useful if the reader is able to calculate and interpret different effect measures, taking into account both the statistical significance and clinical importance of the results.

EFFECT MEASURES

A number of clinically meaningful effect measures have been developed for different types of clinical questions and study designs. These include measures such as the odds ratio (OR), relative risk/risk ratio (RR), relative risk reduction (RRR) and absolute risk reduction (ARR). One increasingly popular measure is the number needed to treat (NNT), which is useful for interpreting results from studies about the effectiveness of a therapy or intervention (DiCenso, 2001). A similar measure is the number needed to harm (NNH) which is used for interpreting the results of prognostic/harm studies. Studies looking at a particular method of diagnosis or assessment often give the results of the test in terms of its sensitivity (proportion of people with a condition who test positively when using the new test) and specificity (proportion of people without the condition who test negatively when using the new test). These results can be converted (using likelihood ratios) into probabilities that express how likely the diagnosis is for a particular patient.

More studies are being published that use these types of measures to report their results, but healthcare practitioners still need to understand how to calculate these themselves. At first some of the calculations may seem a bit intimidating. However, despite their apparent complexity, they usually only involve some simple arithmetic that can, if necessary, be done with pencil and paper. The most effective way of learning these techniques is by working through real examples. The following sections will describe how these measures are calculated and interpreted, along with associated confidence intervals, using as examples results taken from selected papers, including the paper summarized in Box 5.2.

TABLE 5.2 ■ Assessing the Quality of a Study That Investigates Whether a Particular Intervention is Effective: Example Using the CASP Checklist

Type of Question	Assessment Criteria	Response (Yes/Can't Tell/No)	Comment
Screening question	Did the study ask a clearly focused question?	Yes	This study sought to determine the frequency of pressure injuries in acutely ill adults admitted to the ICU and the effect of wearable patient sensors on optimizing care delivery in their prevention.
	Was this a randomized controlled trial (RCT), and was it appropriately so?	Yes	This study compared the frequency of pressure injuries in two groups randomly allocated to wear an electronic sensory monitoring device applied to their chest in either treatment mode (visual warning to turn patient) or control mode (no warning). The study design (RCT) is appropriate for investigating the effectiveness of an intervention.
Detailed question	Were participants appropriately allocated to intervention and control groups?	Can't tell	Although $n = 1564$ patients were assessed for eligibility, of these, 49 did not meet the inclusion criteria, the reasons for not enrolling 203 were not documented, which suggests the possibility of selection bias. The author states that 1312 participants were randomly allocated "by the investigators" to treatment ($n = 659$) or control ($n = 653$) groups using a balanced block design to ensure equal allocation within subgroup strata (ICU unit and treating service team). However, it is not clear who performed the randomization and whether allocation was kept concealed from any of the investigators. Sealed envelopes were used to conceal from the nurses and participants which group the participants were to be allocated to before enrollment.
	Were participants, staff, and study personnel "blind" to the participants' study group?	No	Participants were blinded to which study group they were in, but clinicians and nurses caring for the participants were not. The clinicians were independent to the study team, but it is not clear what the relationship of the study team was to the care staff or whether any of the study team were blinded. It was not possible to blind the nurses after enrollment because for all patients they were required to access a computer in each ICU room and open a monitoring dashboard at the bedside, and for those in the treatment group they received visual warnings if the patient had not been turned according to the established protocol.
	Were all the participants who entered the trial accounted for at its conclusion?	Yes	Yes, the trial profile clearly describes and states intention to treat in the analysis section. Data on all participants originally randomized have been included in the flow diagram and analysis.

Were the participants in all groups followed up and data collected in the same way?	Can't tell	The nurses were trained as to how to use the computer monitoring system and followed established protocols that suggested that participants were followed up in the same way. There were no losses to follow-up as all participants were monitored only while in hospital on the ICU. However, it is unclear what influence the clinical team may have had on data collection because some outcomes were incorrectly reported and resulted in the study being stopped prematurely.
Did the study have enough participants to minimize the play of chance?	No	A power calculation was carried out to detect a 50% difference in the primary outcome measure, hospital-acquired pressure injuries (HAPIs), from 5% in the control group to 2.5% in the intervention group with 80% power, which required 1812 participants. However during the planned interim analysis to check the sample size, the data provided by the clinical team under-reported the number of HAPIs. Because of this error, the study was stopped as the higher sample size required to obtain an increased number of HAPI events was not considered viable. The study ended at 73% recruitment target and was therefore underpowered.
How are the results presented, and what is the main result?		Presented as the percentage of participants experiencing HAPI in each group and compared as an odds ratio. In the treatment mode group, 0.7% (n = 5/659) of participants had pressure injuries compared with 2.3% (15/653) in the control group. The authors conclude that wearing a patient sensor to provide optimal turning is associated with a reduction in pressure injuries (p = 0.031). A significant difference is seen also after adjusting for admitting team, ICU, and risk for pressure injury (p = 0.038).
How precise are the results?		A 95% confidence interval is reported for the odds ratio of 0.33 as (0.12, 0.90), suggesting a reduction in the risk of pressure injuries of between 10% and 88%, but it is unclear whether the results are indicative of clinical significance.
Were all the important outcomes considered so the results can be applied?	No	A number of limitations were addressed in the paper that would need to be considered. In particular, the attention given to these injuries over the past years by Medicaid and the National Quality forum in the US may have influenced practices to reduce injuries before the study began. External validity may have been compromised due to contamination of the control group as this was not a cluster randomized trial of ICU units, but rather individual patients were randomized within ICUs and only the patients were able to be blinded. The clinical importance of the results is also not discussed and the feasibility in terms of extra costs and resources. However the study team took a pragmatic approach that did on the whole deliver useful data on the use of technology in promoting optimal turning practices.

With permission from Critical Appraisal Skills Programme, 2018a. 11 questions to help you make sense of a randomized controlled trial. Available from: <https://casp-uk.net/wp-content/uploads/2018/01/CASP-Randomised-Controlled-Trial-Checklist-2018.pdf>.

Wearable patient sensor	Hospital-acquired pressure injuries		
	Yes	No	Totals
Treatment mode	5 (a)	654 (b)	659
Control mode	15 (c)	638 (d)	653
Totals	20	1292	1312

Fig. 5.3 A 2 × 2 table for interpreting results of a study on the effectiveness of an intervention with data from the study by Pickham et al. (2018) described in Box 5.2.

CALCULATING EFFECT MEASURES FOR TESTING A THERAPY OR INTERVENTION

A 2 × 2 table like the one shown in Fig. 5.3 is a standard tool for calculating clinically meaningful results. Each cell in the table contains a number and is labeled with a letter (a), (b), (c), and (d). In a comparative study participants are divided into two groups: the group that received the "new" or experimental treatment or therapy (cells a and b) and the group that did not (cells c and d). The presence (cells a and c) or absence (cells b and d) of the outcome of interest is reported for both groups. The numbers to go in each cell are obtained from the study results. It is often possible to calculate the numbers if they are not given. Fig. 5.3 uses the results from the study conducted by Pickham et al. (2018) summarized in Box 5.2.

The letters in the cells are used in the formulas for calculating summary measures like the OR, RR, RRR, ARR and NNT. The formulas for calculating these different effect measures are given in Table 5.3. In this section, we will focus specifically on the ARR and the NNT, a popular way of presenting the results of controlled clinical trials. In a trial comparing an experimental treatment with a control treatment, the NNT is the estimated number of patients who need to be treated with the experimental treatment for one additional patient to benefit (Altman, 1998). The smaller the NNT, the more important the treatment effect. In the example (see Box 5.2 and Table 5.3), the ARR is 1.5%, indicating that the absolute benefit of the patient sensor is a 1.5% reduction in the rate of pressure injuries. The NNT is 65 (the figure is typically rounded up toward the more conservative whole number). This means that 65 acutely ill adults need to wear a sensor to prevent one extra patient from developing pressure injuries. When presenting any measure of effect, the 95% confidence interval should also be presented. Box 5.3 demonstrates how the confidence intervals can be calculated for both the ARR and NNT. For the ARR, the 95% confidence interval is 0.2% to 2.9%, indicating that we are 95% certain that the true absolute benefit may be as low as 0.2% or as high as 2.9%. Given that the confidence interval does not include the value of "no effect," we can see that the results are statistically significant. The 95% confidence interval for NNT is 35 to 476. The results suggest that wearing a sensor in intensive care has a small benefit. The benefit is statistically significant but not necessarily clinically important enough to change practice given the additional cost and staff time required.

CALCULATING EFFECT MEASURES FOR ASSESSING THE PERFORMANCE OR ACCURACY OF A DIAGNOSTIC TEST

In a study that tests whether a diagnostic test or assessment works, the new test is compared with an existing "gold standard," which it is assumed diagnoses the target condition with certainty. In the study given in the example in Box 5.4 (van Heyningen et al., 2018), the gold standard is

TABLE 5.3 ■ **Calculating Effects Measures**

Measure	Description	Formula	Example
Odds ratio (OR)	The odds of an event (outcome) in the experimental group divided by the odds of an event in the control group. Usually expressed as a decimal number. An OR of 1 indicates no difference between the two groups (value of "no effect").	$(a/b)/(c/d) =$ ad/bc	$(5/654)/(15/638)$ $= (5 \times 638)/(654 \times 15)$ $= 0.33$
Risk ratio (RR) Also known as relative risk or rate ratio	The risk of an event in the experimental group, known as the experimental event rate (EER) divided by the risk of an event in the control group, known as the control event rate (CER). Usually expressed as a decimal number. A RR of 1 indicates no difference between the two groups.	$(a/(a + b))/(c/(c + d))$	$(5/659)/(15/653)$ $= 0.0076/0.0230$ $= 0.33$
Absolute risk reduction (ARR) Also known as risk difference or rate difference	The risk of an event in the control group (the control event rate [CER]) minus the risk of an event in the experimental group (the experimental event rate [EER]). Usually expressed as a percentage. An ARR of 0% indicates no difference between the two groups.	$c/(c + d) - a/(a + b)$	$(15/653) - (5/659)$ $= 0.0230 - 0.0076$ $= 0.0154 \ (1.54\%)$
Relative risk reduction (RRR)	The ARR divided by the risk of an event in the control group. Can also be calculated as 1 – RR. Usually expressed as a percentage. An RRR of 0 indicates no difference between the two groups.	$ARR/(c/(c + d))$ also $1 - RR$	$0.0154/(15/653)$ or $1 - 0.3304 =$ $0.6696 \ (67\%)$
Number needed to treat (NNT)	The reciprocal of the ARR. Usually expressed as a whole number.	$NNT = 1/ARR$	$1/0.0154 = 65$ (reported as 62 due to rounding errors)

obtained using the Mini-international Neuropsychiatric Interview plus (MINI plus) version 5.0.0. All patients (with and without the condition) receive both the new test and the gold standard test. Fig. 5.4 shows a 2 × 2 table complete with data constructed from the study results. The results of diagnostic studies are usually reported in terms of sensitivity (in our example, this would be the probability of having a positive result using "either screening question plus help question" if you have antenatal depression) and specificity (the probability of having a negative result using "either screening question plus help question" if you do not have antenatal depression). A high sensitivity is a useful result because the presence of a negative test result in a patient virtually rules out a positive diagnosis. In this example (sensitivity 88%), we could say that if Teresa Davies answers "no" to the screening questions plus help question, we can be reasonably sure that she does not have antenatal depression (we would only be wrong in twelve patients out of 100). A high specificity is a useful result because a positive test result in an individual patient effectively rules in

---

BOX 5.3 ■ Calculating 95% Confidence Intervals for the Absolute Risk Reduction and Number Needed to Treat

Formula 95% CI for ARR:
ARR ± 1. 96 √(EER (100 − EER))/(a + b) + (CER (100 − CER))/(c + d)
Example using data from the study by Pickham et al., 2018:
95% CI for ARR = 1.54 ± 1. 96 √(0.76 (100 − 0.76))/659 + 2.30 ((100 − 2.30)/653)
95% CI for ARR = 1.54 ± 1.33% or (0.21, 2.87)%

Formula 95% CI for NNT:
100/upper 95% CI to 100/lower 95% CI of the ARR
Example using data from the study by Pickham et al., 2018:
95% CI for NNT = 100/2.87 to 100/0.21
95% CI for NNT = 35 to 476

BOX 5.4 ■ Example of a Study Assessing the Performance of a Diagnostic Assessment Tool

Scenario

Teresa Davies, a 25-year-old frequent attender at her local health center, visits the practice nurse. She has been pregnant for 6 months, has no mental health problems, but self-reports that she is "feeling down and has a loss of interest." She hardly ever attended the health center until 3 months ago. The nurse feels that Teresa has a 50% chance of having antenatal depression (which means she has a 50% chance of not having antenatal depression) but wants to be more certain before referring her for a specialist assessment. She knows you have recently been on a critical appraisal course and asks you to help her find some more information before deciding what to do. You search on the web and find a paper in PLoS ONE that might be useful.

Clinical Question

In patients with clinical antenatal depression, how accurately does patient response to three simple questions (two screening questions and an additional help question) diagnose clinical antenatal depression?

Evidence

Van Heyningen, T., Honikman, S., Tomlinson, M., Field, S., 2018. Comparison of mental health screening tools for detecting antenatal depression and anxiety disorders in South African women. PLoS ONE 13 (4), e0193697.

Results Reported in the Study

A positive response to "either screening question and the help question" had a sensitivity of 88% (95% CI 81%–95%) and a specificity of 79% (95% CI 74%–84%).

Whooley 2 items + help screening test	MINI Plus diagnosis of antenatal depression		
	Yes	**No**	**Totals**
Yes	72 (a)	63 (b)	135
No	10 (c)	231 (d)	241
Totals	82	294	376

Fig. 5.4 A 2 × 2 table for interpreting results of a study on the accuracy of a diagnostic assessment with data from the study by van Heyningen et al. (2018) described in Box 5.4.

a positive diagnosis. In this example (specificity 79%), if Teresa Davies answers "yes" to either the screening question plus the help question, we could be fairly sure that she had clinical antenatal depression. Twenty-one patients in 100 answer "yes" to one of the questions but do not have clinical antenatal depression. The 95% confidence intervals for sensitivity and specificity given in Box 5.4 suggest that the estimates are fairly precise, with the confidence limits being to within +/− 7% and 5%, respectively. Although the sensitivity and specificity are useful when they are high, it is rare for both the sensitivity and specificity to be high on the same test as there is nearly always a tradeoff between the two.

In addition, the performance of a test is affected by the prevalence of the condition in the underlying population. In an individual patient, this is referred to as the pre-test probability of an individual having the condition. In our scenario, the nurse thought that Teresa Davies had a pre-test probability of 50% of having clinical antenatal depression. What the nurse wants the test to do is to either increase or decrease this probability to indicate more strongly whether she does or does not have antenatal depression, respectively. This is called the *post-test probability.*

In practice what we need to know is, does testing "positive" or "negative" help us to determine whether the patient does or does not have the disease of interest? Technically we can think of this as the likelihood that a positive test result is a true positive and that a negative test result is a true negative. The ratio of true-positive results to false-positive results is known as the *positive likelihood ratio.* The ratio of true-negative results to false-negative results is known as the *negative likelihood ratio.* We can calculate these from the sensitivity and specificity, respectively. The formulas for calculating these measures are given in Table 5.4.

The interpretation of likelihood ratios depends partly on the underlying prevalence (Mant, 2004c). If we convert the prevalence into pre-test odds and multiply the pre-test odds by the negative or positive likelihood ratio, then we can calculate the post-test odds. Most people are more comfortable with using probability than odds, so we can then convert the post-test odds back into a post-test probability of disease. In our scenario, the nurse thought that Teresa Davies had a pre-test probability of 50% of having clinical antenatal depression (and a 50% probability of not having clinical depression). The pre-test probability of 50:50, which is the same as pre-test odds of 1:1, can be combined with the likelihood ratio to give us the post-test odds or probability. In this example, if Teresa screened positive on the test, 1:1 can be multiplied by the likelihood ratio 4.2, giving post-test odds of 4.2:1 in favor of clinical depression. If you are more comfortable with probability than odds, post-test odds of 4.2:1 converts to a more useful, but not diagnostic, post-test probability of 81%. This increase in the probability of antenatal depression after the test suggests that Teresa Davies may well be clinically depressed, and a more detailed assessment by a psychologist may be helpful to firmly establish the correct diagnosis.

TABLE 5.4 ■ **Formulas for Calculating Useful Clinical Measures for Answering Questions About Whether a Particular Diagnostic Test or Method of Assessment Works**

Measure	Formula	Example
Sensitivity	a/(a + c)	72/82 = 0.88 or 88%
Specificity	d/(b + d)	231/294 = 0.79 or 79%
Positive likelihood ratio	Sensitivity/(100 − specificity)	88/(100 − 79) = 4.19
Negative likelihood ratio	(100 − sensitivity)/specificity	(100 − 88)/79 = 0.15
Pre-test odds	Prevalence/100 − prevalence	50/(100 − 50) = 1
Post-test odds	Pre-test odds × likelihood ratio	1 × 4.19 = 4.19
Post-test probability	Post-test odds/(post-test odds + 1)	4.19/(4.19 + 1) = 81%

Note that a simple way of summarizing post-test probabilities for a range of pre-test probabilities and likelihood ratios is by using a special diagram called a *nomogram* (see Straus et al., 2019 for further information).

CALCULATING EFFECT MEASURES FOR PROGNOSTIC STUDIES

Studies of prognosis/harm usually report results in terms of proportions or rates of events in the two groups being compared. If we are satisfied that the evidence from a study is of good enough quality to use, then we need to decide if the association between exposure and outcome is sufficiently strong and convincing for us to have to do something about it. For the scenario given in Box 5.5 related to the paper by Primack et al. (2018), the result of interest is the difference between the initiation rate of traditional cigarette smoking of tobacco in young adults who had previously used e-cigarettes compared with those who had never used e-cigarettes. A 2 × 2 table can be used to aid interpretation of the study results and is given in Fig. 5.5.

BOX 5.5 ■ Example of a Study on Prognosis Assessing the Association between a Smoking Initiation Outcome and Exposure to Risk Factors

Scenario

Lydia Pierce is an 18-year-old girl who enjoys socializing with her friends. Her mother, Jane, is worried because Lydia has started smoking e-cigarettes, which she claims are harmless and that all her friends do it. As Jane's friend, you are also worried and are concerned that there may be future implications for her taking up tobacco smoking. You find a relevant journal article of a recent study carried out at a US school of medicine in Pittsburgh, Pennsylvania.

Clinical Question

Are previously non-smoking young adults who recreationally use e-cigarettes at a higher risk of future initiation of traditional tobacco smoking?

Evidence

Primack, B.A., Shensa, A., Sidani, J.E., Hoffman, B.L., Soneji, S., Sargent, J.D., Hoffman, R., Fine, M.J., 2018. Initiation of traditional cigarette smoking after electronic cigarette smoking among tobacco-naïve US young adults. Am. J. Med. 131, 443.e1–443.e9.

Results Reported in the Study

Young adults who have used e-cigarettes have a fourfold increase in the risk of initiating tobacco smoking within 18 months; that is, 37.5% of young adults who have used e-cigarettes compared with 9% of young adults who have not used e-cigarettes.

Use of e-cigarettes	Initiation of tobacco smoking within 18 months		Totals
	Yes	No	
Yes	6 (a)	10 (b)	16
No	81 (c)	818 (d)	899
Totals	87	828	915

Fig. 5.5 A 2 × 2 table for interpreting results of a study on prognosis/harm with data from the study by Primack et al. (2018) described in Box 5.5.

The researchers did quite appropriately adjust the results for other potential confounding variables such as age, sex, race, and education level, but these results are not shown here. In this example, the absolute risk difference between the two groups is 28.5%, as shown in Table 5.5, with 95% confidence interval 5% to 52%. In general, the research question of the study will determine the importance of the size of the effect measure. For example, if the outcome is mortality, a difference of 5% may be considered sufficient to change practice. If the outcome is benefit obtained by using a very expensive drug with unpleasant side effects, a difference of 5% may not be considered sufficient to change practice. Here, we want to prevent the initiation of tobacco smoking in young adults, and the higher absolute risk difference raises alarm bells about the recreational use of e-cigarettes in previously non-smoking young adults.

Another result not reported in the study is RR (Table 5.5). This measures the relative difference in the percentage initiating cigarette smoking in each group. In this example, the RR tells us that the risk of cigarette smoking is 4.2 times greater among young adults with a previous history of e-cigarette use compared with those with no previous history. As a general rule of thumb, in cohort studies we can say that an RR increase of more than 3 is unlikely to be the result of bias (Straus et al., 2019). From the results of the paper, we can deduce that there is a difference in risk between the two groups and that this difference is unlikely to be the result of bias. But is the difference large enough to convince Lydia to give up using e-cigarettes?

To fully assess the clinical relevance of the findings, we can calculate an additional measure. Table 5.5 shows the formula for calculating the number needed to harm (NNH), for which we first need the absolute risk increase (ARI). The ARI tells us the size of the difference between the two groups, which is 28.5% (or 0.285 from Table 5.5). The ARI in this example tells us that the difference between the groups is equivalent to 285 new tobacco smokers per 1000 young adults. The NNH tells us the number of young adults using e-cigarettes that would have to take place for one extra initiation of tobacco smoking to occur. In the example, the NNH = 4, i.e., not many e-cigarette users at all. In this case, we can conclude that Lydia's e-cigarette use does put her at increased risk of tobacco smoking within 18 months. She should therefore carefully consider the potential consequences of her perceived "as harmless" recreational habits.

P-VALUES AND CONFIDENCE INTERVALS

The way the results of research are reported can often make it difficult to apply them in daily clinical practice. One reason for this is that one of the major concerns of researchers is to establish the likelihood of their result being caused by chance variation. The p-value is frequently presented to illustrate this likelihood. Its value always lies between zero and one. A p-value of 0.5 would tell us that there is a 1 in 2 (50%) probability of observing our data (or data even more extreme) if there is no real effect (i.e., if the null hypothesis is true). If this were the case, we would be unlikely to accept the results of the study as being significant.

TABLE 5.5 ■ Formulas for Calculating Useful Clinical Measures for Answering Questions About Prognosis/Harm

Measure	Formula	Example
Relative risk (RR)	(a/(a + b))/(c/(c + d))	(6/16)/(81/899) = 4.16
Absolute risk difference (increase)	(a/(a + b)) – (c/(c + d))	(6/16) – (81/899) = 0.285
Number needed to harm (NNH)	1/ARI	1/0.285 = 3.5

Conventionally, we accept a p-value of 0.05 or below as being statistically significant. That means that a significant result could occur 5 times in 100 (or 1 time in 20) when, in fact, there is really no difference between the groups being compared. Some papers may use a more rigorous cutoff point of p equal to 0.01 or below as statistically significant (a 1 in 100 probability). The p-value alone does not give any indication of the size or direction of the difference (or treatment effect) (Altman et al., 2000). Therefore it does not help you assess what the likely effect will be on your patient.

Health-related research studies should present results accompanied by confidence intervals, which provide more information than the p-value alone. A formal definition of a confidence interval is "a range of values for a variable of interest constructed so that this range has a specified probability of including the true value of the variable" (Porta, 2014). The accepted convention is to use the 95% confidence interval. This means that you can be 95% certain that the true value of the variable of interest lies within the upper and lower limits of the confidence interval.

Confidence intervals are a clinically useful way of measuring the precision of an estimate of effect size. When evaluating the effect of an intervention, a confidence interval not only provides us with information on statistical significance, but also indicates with a certain degree of confidence (e.g., 95% or 95 times out of 100) the range within which the true treatment effect is likely to lie. If, when comparing interventions, the confidence interval includes the value of "no effect," then the difference between the two intervention groups is not statistically significant. The narrower the gap between the upper and lower 95% confidence interval limits, the more certain we will be about the precision of the estimate. The 95% confidence interval can be calculated for most common statistical estimates.

Can I Apply the Results in My Clinical Setting?

So far we have dealt with the quality of health-related research studies—how well has a study been conducted for the research question being asked, and how to calculate and interpret the results. But can we trust the study's results enough to apply them in our own clinical setting? What needs to be recognized here is that not all high-quality studies are applicable to all patients or all clinical settings. Health-related research takes place all over the world, in settings that may be very different from the one in which your patients are found. In addition, there is a tendency for studies to include "scientifically clean" populations (Greenhalgh, 2014), excluding patients who have co-existing illnesses or additional risk factors. This can mean that patients included in health-related research are often very different from those seen in everyday clinical practice. The context in which you practice and/or the context in which each patient's consultation takes place is, to some degree, unique. Alongside the assessment of a study's quality, it is important to consider whether the results obtained can be applied to your patient's and your clinical setting. Can the results of a trial recruiting patients 18 to 50 years of age be applied to patients over 60 years of age? If a study has been conducted in Brazil, what do the results mean with regard to patients being treated in the UK?

It is unlikely that the patients and settings used in a research study will ever be identical to yours. When addressing the issue of applicability, we need to consider the extent to which differences in patients and settings might affect the results. Are the differences so great that we might expect the direction of effect to alter? If the differences would only change the size or extent of the effect of the treatment, rather than changing the effect from one of benefit to one of harm, then it may be possible to adjust the result to reflect the impact in your patients. For example, if a treatment has been shown to be effective on a relatively fit study population, we might expect a greater effect to be observed on a very sick patient seen in practice. Similarly if a diagnostic test was assessed using a hospital population, would it still be applicable in general practice?

QUESTIONS FOR ASSESSING APPLICABILITY

The assessment of both quality and applicability can be used to determine whether a study is worth reading in full. If a fundamental flaw is identified in the study design that means the results of the study cannot be trusted, there is little point in reading the full article. Similarly, if it is clear from the details presented in the study that the results cannot be applied to your patient population and/or the clinical setting, then there is no need to read further.

The assessment of applicability is not an exact science and requires some degree of subjectivity. Specific questions can help to ascertain the applicability of a study's results. Unlike the quality assessment, the same questions can be used whatever type of question or study design is being appraised. Questions to consider when assessing applicability include the following:

- **What are the characteristics of the participants in the study?** Do they differ from the patients you see in practice? If so, do they differ on factors that could potentially affect the outcome of interest (consider age, co-morbidity, severity of condition, gender, and so on). Are the differences likely to affect the direction of the effect seen in the study or just the size of the effect?

- **Where has the study been conducted?** Is the study setting so different from yours that the results achieved in the study are unlikely to be achieved in your clinical setting? Again, are the differences likely to affect the direction of the effect seen in the study or just the magnitude of the effect?

- **Is it feasible to introduce the intervention or test described in the study?** Suppose the results of a research study into the care of patients with stroke suggest that patient outcomes are better when they are looked after in a specialist unit (i.e., one that requires certain types of equipment and staff with specialist training) rather than in a general ward. Such a change may not be possible on your unit. This does not mean that you should give up altogether (the issue should perhaps be referred to your unit manager); however, it does mean that you will need to look at other aspects of stroke management that are within the capacity of your team to deliver.

- **Have all the important outcomes been considered?** Have the researchers considered all the outcomes that are truly important to the patient and all those involved in their care and treatment planning? If not, how does this affect the interpretation of the results presented? Researchers often focus on outcome measures that are relatively quick and easy to measure, rather than those that are of practical importance. For example, surrogate outcomes, such as blood pressure, are often used to reflect the more clinically important "hard" outcomes, such as risk of heart attack or death. Surrogate outcomes are often used when the observation of a clinical outcome would require a long follow-up. However, when interpreting the findings from surrogate outcomes, we have to be certain of the link between the surrogate and clinical outcome and whether its utility is well established.

- **Do any reported benefits outweigh the costs?** When thinking of the costs and benefits of the intervention or test, think beyond purely financial terms. In most situations, doing something new or in a different way will involve stopping doing something else. The costs of "stopping" need to be weighed against the benefits of the proposed change. Where the costs are perceived by the patient and/or staff as being too high, the proposed change is unlikely to be accepted.

- **What are your patient's preferences?** Incorporating research evidence into practice should not mean ignoring patient preference. All patients are different, and what one patient considers a reasonable intervention, treatment plan, or outcome may be unacceptable to another. Forcing a patient to use the intervention indicated by evidence would be unethical and may be counterproductive.

Exercise

We encourage you to consolidate your learning by undertaking the two exercises on the website.

Summary

In this chapter, we have established why critical appraisal is necessary and important for evidence-based practice. The key principles of research design underpinning the assessment of a study have been outlined. Critical appraisal for evidence-based practice is a three-part process comprising assessment of the quality of the study, interpretation of the results, and assessment of the applicability of the findings to the patients in your setting. We have seen that it would be unrealistic to expect to find perfect research studies that match exactly a certain clinical context; the idea is to identify studies that can be applied to a specific context where the design is *good enough* for the results to be trusted. This chapter has provided examples of how this can be done for three different types of clinical question that require the use of different research designs. It is important to recognize that all three aspects of the critical appraisal process are interlinked. The quality and applicability aspects are probably the most important parts of critical appraisal to learn. Only you know the setting in which you wish to apply the results, and published studies very rarely assess their own quality, but it is becoming more common to publish study results in clinically useful forms. Chapter 9 describes how to use research evidence to inform clinical decisions for individual patients.

The tools in this chapter contain the basic questions necessary for assessing the quality of research studies in the practice environment. More sophisticated critical appraisal tools and techniques are available for people who are becoming more experienced or are doing critical appraisal on questions not covered in this chapter such as economic evaluations (Dumville and Soares, 2009; Greenhalgh, 2014). Presenting the results of critical appraisal to colleagues in a systematic way, making explicit the process used to come to these conclusions, is an important part of preparing for change (Melnyk, 2014). The critical appraisal tools mentioned earlier provide a method for generating a summary of a study. The Centre for Evidence-Based Medicine in Oxford also produces CATmaker software, which is a computer program that can be used to make numerical summaries. Raw data from the study can be entered into the program to calculate some useful numbers for summarizing the results in terms of effects on individual patients (e.g., the NNT).

It is important to recognize that critical appraisal is only one part of the evidence-based process and on its own will not result in improvements in the quality of care that you might want to achieve. It is therefore important that you take equal care to learn and practice the other stages in the process described in the other chapters of this manual.

Acknowledgements

We give special thanks to Mark Newman, Tony Roberts, Faith Gibson, and Anne-Marie Glenny, whose contributions to previous editions have provided the foundation for this chapter.

References

Altman, D.G., 1998. Confidence intervals for the number needed to treat. Br. Med. J. 317, 1309–1312.

Altman, D.G., Machin, D., Bryant, T.N., Gardner, M.J., 2000. Statistics with Confidence: Confidence Intervals and Statistical Guidelines, second ed. BMJ Publishing: London.

Blaikie, N., 2009. Designing Social Research, second ed. Polity Press: Cambridge.

Bowling, A., 2014. Research Methods in Health: Investigating Health and Health Services, fourth ed. Open University Press: Maidenhead.

Critical Appraisal Skills Programme, 2018a. 11 questions to help you make sense of a randomised controlled trial. Available from: <https://casp-uk.net/wp-content/uploads/2018/01/CASP-Randomised-Controlled-Trial-Checklist-2018.pdf> (Accessed 27.04.19).

Critical Appraisal Skills Programme, 2018b. 12 questions to help you make sense of a diagnostic test study. Available from: <https://casp-uk.net/wp-content/uploads/2018/01/CASP-Diagnostic-Checklist-2018.pdf> (Accessed 27.04.19).

Critical Appraisal Skills Programme, 2018c. 12 questions to help you make sense of a cohort study. Available from: <https://casp-uk.net/wp-content/uploads/2018/01/CASP-Cohort-Study-Checklist_2018.pdf> (Accessed 27.04.19).

DiCenso, A., 2001. Clinically useful measures of the effects of treatment. Evid. Based Nurs. 4, 36–39.

Dumville, J., Soares, M., 2009. The economics of clinical decision making. In: Thompson, C., Dowding, D. (Eds.), Essential Decision Making and Clinical Judgement for Nurses. Churchill Livingstone: London, pp. 197–216.

Egger, M., Davey-Smith, G., Altman, D.G., 2001. Systematic reviews in healthcare, second ed. BMJ Publishing: London.

Evans, D., Pearson, A., 2001. Systematic reviews: gatekeepers of nursing knowledge. J. Clin. Nurs. 10, 593–599.

Faraoni, D., Schaefer, S.T., 2016. Randomized controlled trials vs. observational studies: why not just live together? BMC Anesthesiol. 16 (1), 102.

French, P., 2002. What is the evidence on evidence-based nursing? An epistemological concern. J. Adv. Nurs. 37 (3), 250–257.

Gray, J.A.M., 2009. Evidence-Based Health-Care and Public Health: How to Make Decisions About Health Services and Public Health, third ed. Churchill Livingstone: Edinburgh.

Gray, J.R., Grove, S.K., Sutherland, S., 2016. Burns and Grove's The Practice of Nursing Research: Appraisal, Synthesis, and Generation of Evidence, eighth ed. Saunders: Philadelphia.

Greenhalgh, T., 2014. How to Read a Paper: The basics of Evidence-Based Medicine, fifth ed. John Wiley and Sons: Chichester, West Sussex.

Guyatt, G., Rennie, D., Meade, M.O., Cook, D.J., 2014. Users' Guides to the Medical Literature. Essentials of Evidence-Based Clinical Practice, third ed. McGraw-Hill Education: New York.

Guyatt, G., Rennie, D., Meade, M.O., Cook, D.J., 2015. Users' Guides to the Medical Literature: a Manual for Evidence-Based Clinical Practice, third ed. McGraw-Hill: New York.

Kirkwood, B.R., Sterne, J.A.C., 2003. Essentials of Medical Statistics, second ed. Wiley Blackwell: Oxford.

Lijmer, J.G., Mol, B.W., Heisterkamp, S., Bonsel, G.J., Prins, M.H., van der Meulen, J.H., et al., 1999. Empirical evidence of design-related bias in studies of diagnostic tests. J. Am. Med. Assoc. 282 (11), 1061–1066.

Malone, H., Nicholl, H., Tracey, C., 2014. Awareness and minimisation of systematic bias in research. Br. J. Nurs. 23 (5), 279–282.

Mant, J., 2004a. Studies assessing diagnostic tests. In: Dawes, M., Davies, P., Gray, A., Mant, J., Seers, J., Snowball, R. (Eds.), Evidence-Based Practice: A Primer for Health-Care Professionals, second ed. Churchill Livingstone: London, pp. 67–78.

Mant, J., 2004b. Case control studies. In: Dawes, M., Davies, P., Gray, A., Mant, J., Seers, J., Snowball, R. (Eds.), Evidence-Based Practice: a Primer for Health-Care Professionals, second ed. Churchill Livingstone: London, pp. 83–100.

Mant, J., 2004c. Is this test effective? In: Dawes, M., Davies, P., Gray, A., Mant, J., Seers, J., Snowball, R. (Eds.), Evidence-Based Practice: A Primer for Health Care Professionals, second ed. Churchill Livingstone: London, pp. 153–180.

Matthews, J.N.S., 2006. An introduction to randomized controlled clinical trials, second ed. Chapman & Hall/CRC: Boca Raton.

Melnyk, B.M., 2014. Creating a vision and motivating a change to evidence-based practice in individuals, teams and organizations. In: Melnyk, B.M., Fineout-Overholt, E. (Eds.), Evidence-Based Practice in Nursing and Healthcare: A Guide to Best Practice, third ed. Lippincott: Philadelphia, pp. 316–329.

O'Mathuna, D.P., Fineout-Overholt, E., 2014. Critically appraising quantitative evidence for clinical decision making. In: Melnyk, B.M., Fineout-Overholt, E. (Eds.), Evidence-based practice in nursing and healthcare: a guide to best practice, third ed. Lippincott, Philadelphia, pp. 87–138.

Oxman, A.D., Sackett, D.L., Guyatt, G.H., et al., 1993. Users' Guides to the Medical Literature. I. How to get started. JAMA 270 (17), 2093–2095.

Pickham, D., Berte, N., Pihulic, A., Valdez, A., Mayer, B., 2018. Effect of a wearable patient sensor on care delivery for preventing pressure injuries in acutely ill adults: a pragmatic randomized clinical trial (LS-HAPI study). Int. J. Nurs. Stud. 80, 12–19.

Porta, M., 2014. A Dictionary of Epidemiology, sixth ed. Oxford University Press: Oxford.

Primack, B.A., Shensa, A., Sidani, J.E., Hoffman, B.L., Soneji, S., Sargent, J.D., et al., 2018. Initiation of traditional cigarette smoking after electronic cigarette smoking among tobacco-naïve US young adults. Am. J. Med. 131 (4), 443.e1–443.e9.

Straus, S., Glaziou, P., Richardson, W.S., Haynes, R.B., 2019. Evidence-Based Medicine: How to Practice and Teach EBM, fifth ed. Elsevier: Edinburgh.

Sim, J., Wright, C., 2000. Basic elements of research design. In: Sim, J., Wright, C. (Eds.), Research in Health-Care: Concepts, Designs and Methods. Nelson Thornes: Cheltenham.

Stevens, K.R., 2014. Critically appraising knowledge for clinical decision making. In: Melnyk, B.M., Fineout-Overholt, E. (Eds.), Evidence-Based Practice in Nursing and Health-Care: a Guide to Best Practice, third ed. Lippincott: Philadelphia, pp. 77–86.

Summerskill, W.S.M., 2001. Hierarchy of evidence. In: McGovern, D.B.P., Valori, R.M., Summerskill, W.S.M., Levi, M. (Eds.), Key Topics in Evidence-Based Medicine. BIOS Scientific Publishers: Oxford, pp. 14–16.

Van Heyningen, T., Honikman, S., Tomlinson, M., Field, S., 2018. Comparison of mental health screening tools for detecting antenatal depression and anxiety disorders in South African women. PLoS ONE 13 (4), e0193697.

Further Reading

Internet Resources

There are numerous websites that contain materials for critical appraisal. However, these sites often change their website address, and new sites are opening up all the time. The Centre for Evidence-Based Medicine at Oxford has a number of useful resources found at www.cebm.net as does www.jamaevidence.com, but the latter requires a subscription.

Books

Crombie, I.K., 1996. The Pocket Guide to Critical Appraisal. BMJ Publishing: London.

Greenhalgh, T., 2014. How to Read a Paper: The basics of Evidence-Based Medicine, fifth ed. John Wiley and Sons: Chichester.

Greenhalgh, T., 2017. How to Implement Evidence-Based Healthcare. John Wiley and Sons: Chichester.

Melnyk, B.M., Fineout-Overholt, E., 2014. Evidence-Based Practice in Nursing and Health-Care: a Guide to Best Practice, third ed. Lippincott: Philadelphia.

Ogier, M.E., 2002. Reading Research: How to Make Research More Approachable, third ed. Baillière Tindall: London.

Straus, S., Glaziou, P., Richardson, W.S., Haynes, R.B., 2019. Evidence-Based Medicine: How to Practice and Teach EBM, fifth ed. Elsevier: Edinburgh.5—Using Evidence from Quantitative Studies.

CHAPTER 6

Using Evidence from Mixed Methods Studies

Diane Bunn ■ Sarah Hanson

KEY POINTS

■ Mixed methods research (MMR) is an emerging methodology.

■ MMR encompasses *both* quantitative and qualitative research methods in a single study, or program of inquiry, designed to address research questions or complex phenomena that cannot be answered solely by using quantitative or qualitative methods.

■ MMR is distinct from multi-methods research, as multi-methods research uses one or more methods of data collection within *either* a quantitative *or* a qualitative paradigm.

■ The defining feature of MMR is the intentional integration, using appropriate methods, at any of the three stages in the research process: design, methods and interpretation.

■ Process evaluations assess fidelity—the extent to which a program is operating as it was intended. They are designed to understand whether an intervention works and in what context, rather than only focusing on statistical and/or clinical significance in numerical outcomes. Typically, they will use both quantitative and qualitative data as complementary information to give a much broader perspective.

■ As MMR addresses complex healthcare questions, research using this methodology is likely to be highly relevant for nurses, and thus nurses need an understanding of the quality of the research. As an emerging methodology, there are currently no substantive critical appraisal tools for MMR, but there are a number of fundamental criteria that MMR should address, which we describe here.

Introduction

This chapter focuses on mixed methods research (MMR), and its contribution to evidence-based health care. We will define the term *mixed methods research* and describe the nature of mixed methods inquiry as an appropriate methodology to address complex research questions. We will present the different ways MMR is conducted, as well as discussing methods of critically evaluating MMR studies, and how to apply findings to clinical practice. To consolidate learning, we have provided examples.

A mixed methods approach encompasses both quantitative and qualitative research methods in a single study, or program of inquiry, designed to address research questions or complex phenomena that cannot be answered solely by using quantitative or qualitative methods (Heyvaert et al., 2013). MMR is more than simply collecting both qualitative and quantitative data and combining the findings; it is the intentional integration, using appropriate methods, at any of the three stages in the research process: design, methods, and interpretation (Fetters and Molina-Azorin, 2017).

The central premise behind MMR is that by combining and integrating data, additional breadth, depth, and a more diverse perspective is attained (Ozawa and Pongpirul, 2014), providing a greater understanding of the phenomenon than the individual component studies. In other words, the whole is greater than the sum of the parts (Creswell, 2015; Bryman, 2007; Fetters et al., 2013). As such, the strengths of various methodological approaches are used to address complex research questions providing flexibility and a multi-dimensional view when answering the complex research questions found in health care (Burke Johnson and Onwuegbuzie, 2004; Mason 2006).

As MMR crosses the boundaries of both quantitative and qualitative methodologies, the philosophical underpinnings of MMR have generated considerable debate. Creswell describes the philosophical stance of MMR as being that of pragmatism, or very simply as "what works"(Creswell et al., 2011). Our intention in this chapter is not to comment on this debate, rather to help you appraise and use MMR studies. For those of you who would like further understanding of the discussions on the philosophical perspectives relating to MMR as an independent methodology, we recommend further reading by some of the leading proponents (see Further Reading at the end of this chapter).

MMR should not be confused with multi-method research in which multiple methods within a single quantitative or qualitative paradigm are used (Shorten and Smith, 2017; Fetters and Molina-Azorin, 2017). For example, where a combination of interviews, focus groups, and documentary analysis have been used within a qualitative study, this would be described as multi-methods research, rather than MMR. Similarly, when a qualitative design and method have been used to collect and analyze some quantitative data, but a rigorous quantitative approach has not been followed, this would be seen as multi-methods research. Another example of this would be a survey in which respondents are asked to indicate an answer from the categories provided, as well as provide free-text comments that are analyzed separately (Pluye and Hong, 2014).

What Is Mixed Methods Research?

MMR, together with quantitative (Chapter 4) and qualitative (Chapter 5) research, are the three major research paradigms in health care. MMR is the most recent development arising from the need for innovative approaches to investigate the increasing complexities inherent in current healthcare research (Fetters et al., 2013). By complexity, we mean to include the complex needs of patients and their families; the complexity of any intervention that is being evaluated; and also the complex interplay of individual characteristics, social determinants, and healthcare delivery systems (Guise et al., 2017). These challenges require a multidimensional research approach to capture inherent complexity. Whereas quantitative research provides measurable evidence, helping to establish cause and effect, qualitative research provides context, meaning and experiential evidence, so that when both qualitative and quantitative findings are combined and integrated, as in MMR, this process maximizes the strength of each.MMR designs are very well suited to this and are likely to be more appropriate than making a dichotomous choice between quantitative and qualitative methods.

In healthcare, researchers and healthcare providers need to understand why differences occur between populations regarding certain health issues such as differing treatment effects, adherence to treatment, and behavioral factors that influence health and disability. MMR, by encouraging inter-disciplinary working, allows researchers to view problems from multiple perspectives, contextualize information, develop a more complete understanding of a problem, triangulate results, quantify hard-to-measure constructs, examine processes/experiences along with outcomes, and thus capture a macro picture of an issue (Creswell et al., 2011). Creswell, a proponent of MMR, maintains that patients' viewpoints, together with cultural and social factors are fundamental to determining the effectiveness of healthcare, as they provide the context within which healthcare operates (Creswell et al., 2011). As such, the resultant findings may be more beneficial for consumers of research. For example, commissioners may want numerical, quantitative outcomes (such as "How many?"), whereas users (patients, carers, health professionals) may be more concerned with their healthcare experience.

While recognizing the contribution that MMR can make to healthcare research, the disadvantages of MMR are the increased complexity of the data, the additional integration steps needed, and dealing with contradictions in the data. Thus more resources are often required in terms of time, personnel, training, and expertise (Shorten and Smith, 2017).

PROCESS EVALUATION

Typically, process evaluations that often run in parallel with a research trial, use mixed methods. Process evaluations are designed to understand how an intervention works, and in what context, rather than only focusing on statistical and/or clinical significance in numerical outcomes. As such, they will use both quantitative and qualitative data as complementary information to give a much broader perspective. Broadly, a process evaluation assesses fidelity—the extent to which a program is operating as it was intended and the contextual factors that influence how the intervention is implemented (U.S. Government Accountability Office, 2011). For example, an RCT will measure effect size, or other statistical measure of change and at the end of a trial the treatment or intervention may be recommended to policy makers or practitioners. However, these results might not give us the full picture or detect the more subtle nuances that affected implementation. In complex public health interventions, you may also wish to measure the quality of your program implementation: its dose; reach; recruitment; sustainability and context; and how these elements have affected its impact (Centers for Disease Control and Prevention, 2008; Steckler and Linnan, 2002). In both scenarios, a process evaluation designed using mixed methods would examine processes, context, and experiences as well as outcomes (Plano Clark, 2010). The aim is to understand the mechanisms of change and any interacting components and to build a theoretical understanding. For example, in a research trial the outcomes and results may not tell us whether the intervention was delivered as intended; whether the whole package or only parts of it were necessary to deliver the outcome; whether different sub-groups responded differently; or whether the intervention would work in the "real world" or in another context. This is where a process evaluation is vitally important as it seeks to provide additional data to help explain the results (O'Cathain et al., 2013).

An example could be research investigating whether nurse consultations using a behavioral intervention to promote physical activity and reduce weight for overweight patients with type 2 diabetes have positive outcomes. The outcome evaluation would assess whether this had been achieved. The process evaluation would assess *how* this had been achieved. This would likely include recorded interviews between the patient and nurse to assess fidelity (or adaptions) to the protocol. This is important because interventions often have better effects when delivered with high fidelity (Dane and Schneider, 1998). These data would be analyzed both quantitatively (minutes spent in consultation, adherence to the protocol) and qualitatively (adaptions and responses made). It could also include daily diaries in which the patient self-reported food intake and physical activity that would be quantified. Finally, qualitative data from interviews with both the patient and nurse would aim to elucidate their perceptions of the program and better understand mechanisms of action, mediators of behavioral change, and contextual factors. Each data set would be analyzed and findings triangulated, thus strengthening the findings. Indeed the advantage is the combination of the strengths of each method to answer the research question. This is thus a pragmatic approach to knowledge generation (both theory and practice) that considers multiple perspectives and standpoints (Burke Johnson et al., 2007). The results thus have the potential to give a more complete understanding than would have been provided by each data set alone (Creswell 2015).

For further information on process evaluation in public health, see the Centers for Disease Control and Prevention webpages (Centers for Disease Control and Prevention, 2008).

Role of Mixed Methods Research in Evidence-Based Practice

Nurses are increasingly expected to ensure that their practice is evidence-based. Evidence-based practice (EBP) was pioneered by David Sacket, an American-Canadian doctor, who recognized the value and benefit to patients of ensuring that the best research evidence, when integrated with clinical expertise and patient values improves outcomes (Sackett et al., 2000). In other words, as an internationally recognized quantitative researcher with expertise in developing and refining quantitative research methods, he recognized that EBP was more than the application of numerical findings; it was also contextual. The integration of numerical and contextual data is the basis of MMR, which is designed to address the complexities of healthcare research.

Mixed Methods Research Methods

In MMR, research questions should indicate that a mixed methods approach is the appropriate methodology to address the question. For example, in the study by Desborough et al., the overarching research question developed to drive the study was:

> *"What is the relationship of general (family) practice characteristics and nurse consultation characteristics to patient satisfaction and enablement arising from general (family) practice nursing care?"*
> (DESBOROUGH ET AL., 2018.)

Similarly, Greenwood and Habibi investigated the benefits of a mentoring service for informal carers. They commenced their mixed methods study with quantitative and qualitative questions and then developed a final question:

> *"What mechanisms can be proposed to understand how mentoring may work (integrating quantitative and qualitative findings)?"*
> (GREENWOOD AND HABIBI, 2014)

As integration of quantitative and qualitative paradigms is the defining feature of MMR, the three points of integration: study design, study methods (data collection and analysis), and data interpretation and reporting need careful consideration. These are discussed more fully in the following sections.

INTEGRATION AT STUDY DESIGN LEVEL

Creswell described two overarching study designs for MMR: "basic," which can be subdivided further into convergent parallel, explanatory sequential and exploratory sequential designs (Table 6.1), and "advanced," which also incorporate embedded, transformative, or multiphase designs. All MMR will fall into one of the basic study designs, whereas the advanced study designs relate to an additional level or levels of interplay between qualitative and quantitative studies (Creswell, 2015). It is worth noting that in each study design type (whether basic or advanced), the qualitative and quantitative types may have different weighting and dominance, and this can also vary during the course of the studies. For this chapter, we have focused on the basic study designs as these are increasingly accepted practice in what is a developing methodological field. For information on advanced study designs (embedded, transformative, and multiphase), please refer to Creswell's text (Creswell, 2015). The three basic study designs areas follows:

1. Convergent parallel

   This is when both qualitative and quantitative studies are conducted separately, in parallel, but may not be completely integrated until the analysis stage.

TABLE 6.1 ■ Sequence of Quantitative and Qualitative Studies in a Basic Study Design

Study Design	Quantitative	Qualitative	Sequence
Convergent parallel	First	First	Quantitative and qualitative studies conducted in parallel
Explanatory sequential	First	Second	Quantitative study done initially, followed by qualitative study
Exploratory sequential	Second	First	Qualitative study done initially, followed by quantitative study

An example of a convergent parallel design was the study conducted by Ankuda et al. in which quantitative and qualitative data were collected concurrently to investigate which elements of a hospital at home service make the most difference to patients receiving palliative care (Ankuda et al., 2018).

2. Explanatory sequential

The quantitative study is undertaken initially, data are analyzed, and this is followed by a qualitative study that explains the quantitative results in more depth.

An example of an explanatory sequential study design is an investigation of nurses' perspectives of a new care intervention for patients with COPD in primary care, in which quantitative questionnaire data were collected preintervention and post-intervention and then qualitative focus groups conducted to explore previous findings (Weldam et al., 2017).

3. Exploratory sequential

The initial study is qualitative, often used to explore a phenomenon in which there is little understanding to inform and develop a second, quantitative study. An example of this was a study exploring self-disclosure of mental health issues in which participants took part in interviews or focus groups, and, based on these findings and a literature review, an anonymous online survey was developed and distributed (Marino et al., 2016).

INTEGRATION AT THE METHODS LEVEL (SAMPLING, DATA COLLECTION AND DATA ANALYSIS)

Integration at the methods level occurs through the linking of the methods during sampling, data collection, and analysis. The usual methods of sampling in quantitative and qualitative studies are probability and purposive, respectively (see Chapters 4 and 5). In MMR, both methods can be used, but it is the way they are linked with the overall research that is the defining feature. Fetters and Molina-Azorin describe four strategies: identical, separate, nested, and multi-level. In an identical strategy, both quantitative and qualitative data are collected from the entire study sample, in contrast to a separate strategy in which the opposite occurs—data are collected from two separate samples. In a nested strategy, data are collected from a subset of the entire study sample, and in multi-level strategies, data are collected from multiple subsets (Fetters and Molina-Azorin, 2017). For example, when investigating the health benefits of walking groups, Hanson et al. recruited two groups of people: stakeholders responsible for setting up and managing the scheme and volunteer Walking Champions who led the walks (Hanson et al., 2016).

Integration in data analysis in MMR refers to the way in which both types of data relate to each other (Onwuegbuzie et al., 2007). A number of typologies have been described (e.g.,

Onwuegbuzie et al., 2007; Fetters et al., 2013; Fetters and Molina-Azorin, 2017; O'Cathain et al., 2010), but essentially they fall into four main types:

1. Data from each study are analyzed separately, and integration occurs as a subsequent step. This is common in convergent parallel study designs. A number of strategies have been described to achieve this, such as visual representations or displays of data in tables, matrices, or graphs (Fetters and Molina-Azorin, 2017). An example of this can be found in the study by Beck et al. in their investigation of stress in nurses working in pediatric intensive care units (Beck et al., 2017).

2. In sequential study designs (exploratory or explanatory), the data analysis of the initial study informs the development of the subsequent study or studies.

3. Data from all the component studies are analyzed concurrently with the researchers "following a thread." After an initial analysis of both studies, key themes are selected and followed as they "thread" across the component studies. O'Cathain et al. cite an example in health services research in which the theme of "self-rationing" in relation to health service use was identified early in the research process, so it was tracked across all the findings from each of the component studies (O'Cathain et al., 2010).

4. Data from either the quantitative or qualitative study are transformed to qualitative or quantitative (respectively). For example qualitative data may be analyzed using content analysis, to provide numerical findings, or quantitative findings may be described narratively and integrated with the narrative findings from the qualitative study.

INTEGRATION AT THE DATA INTERPRETATION AND REPORTING STAGE

Integration at the data interpretation and reporting stage is probably the most challenging stage and is perhaps the reason why there is a tendency to report findings from the qualitative and quantitative studies separately, as stand-alone studies in different publications, but this undermines the aim of MMR. In MMR, meta-inferences are made based on the interpretation of the data from the component studies when seen as a whole. Using defined methods for data integration and interpretation ensures credibility of the findings (Farquhar et al., 2011).

Fetters and Molina-Azorin describe how MMR researchers should interpret the data, looking at the degree of coherence between the qualitative and quantitative data types (Fetters and Molina-Azorin, 2017). Conclusions may be based on four possibilities: confirmation, complementarity, expansion, or discordance. Confirmation is when the data confirm the results of each other, with similar conclusions. Complementarity occurs when the data provide different, but complementary conclusions. Expansion is when the integrated data provides depth or breadth beyond the component studies, and discordance occurs when qualitative and quantitative findings are inconsistent, incongruous, contradictory, or conflicting.

Discordance in findings are not necessarily a problem. In fact, such findings could be seen as justification of using MMR, because of the way in which MMR provides multiple perspectives, with the possibility that discordant findings may help to improve the problem analysis and pave the way for further investigation. Moffat et al. (2006) outlined six strategies for managing and investigating how discrepancies in data should be managed, drawing on their work that evaluated the impact of welfare rights advice on health and social outcomes in people aged over 60 years. They found that that there was a discrepancy between the quantitative findings, which demonstrated little effect of the intervention, and the qualitative findings, which suggested wide-ranging benefits. To explain this discordance, they suggested that the study design, methods, and analyses should be re-examined, focusing on six areas: whether the two study designs were investigating different issues, what was the methodological rigor of the component studies, whether the samples and data were comparable, whether additional data were needed, whether the intervention had worked as expected, and whether the outcomes of the two components matched (Moffatt et al., 2006).

Appraising and Reporting Mixed Methods Research

Critical appraisal tools are an integral process in evidence-based practice because they enable consumers (practitioners, researchers, commissioners, and patients) to make informed decisions about the quality of the research and its applicability to practice (see Chapters 4 and 5). Similarly, reporting guidelines ensure that key aspects of studies are reported.

As an emergent methodology, guidelines against which to appraise the quality of MMR are needed for judging the quality of MMR, as MMR has a number of unique features that should be appraised according to its own set of quality criteria (Fàbregues and Molina-Azorín, 2017). There are currently no universally agreed critical appraisal or reporting criteria (Creswell, 2015; Fàbregues and Molina-Azorín, 2017), although there are a number of developments aiming to address this deficit. Overall, there appears to be some agreement about the range of criteria that need to be included in an MMR-specific critical appraisal framework, but definitions need to be agreed on and evidence provided regarding the framework's psychometric properties (O'Cathain et al., 2008; Heyvaert et al., 2013; Beck and Harrison, 2016).

In 2011, Creswell et al. were commissioned by the Office of Behavioral and Social Sciences Research to provide a resource providing guidance to NIH investigators on how to rigorously develop and evaluate MMR applications (Creswell et al., 2011). Drawing on their own work, as well as that of O'Cathain et al. (O'Cathain et al., 2010) and Schifferdecker and Reed (Schifferdecker and Reed 2009), they provided criteria against which to judge the quality of the applications. These included specific funder requirements (such as quality of institutional support, innovation) as well as specific criteria relating to the conduct of the mixed methods studies themselves (Box 6.1).

Subsequently, a systematic review identified thirteen critical appraisal frameworks for appraising MMR, reporting that there were substantial variations in their content and construction. In their analysis, Heyvaert et al. generated 13 broad domains that had been addressed within the frameworks to varying degrees (Box 6.2). The authors concluded that there was a lack of consensus for an agreed tool, but as critical appraisal frameworks are favored by funding bodies, journal editors, researchers, and practitioners, there is a need (Heyvaert et al., 2013).

BOX 6.1 ■ Criterion Relating Specifically to Mixed Methods Research Design When Appraising Funding Applications

- Is there a description of the philosophy or theory informing the research and the ways this philosophy or theory shapes the investigation?
- Have the applicants offered a convincing explanation of why mixed methods research is needed to address the study aims and the value added by using this approach (e.g., explained how alternative designs would be inappropriate or inadequate)?
- Is there a clear description of the full study design, including where integration occurs (e.g., using a comprehensive figure or matrix)?
- Is the integration of the methods well described, including the timing, techniques, and responsibilities for integration?
- Is the design appropriate for the study aims?
- Are the methods consistent with established standards of rigor for quantitative and qualitative data collection and analysis (e.g., sampling, sample size, and analysis plans are specified for each method, with appropriate citations)?

From Creswell, J.W., Klassen, A.C., Plano Clark, V.L., Smith, K.C. 2011. Best Practices for Mixed Methods Research in the Health Sciences. Washington, D.C.: Office of Behavioral and Social Sciences Research, National Institutes of Health.

BOX 6.2 ■ Criteria for Critical Appraisal of Mixed Methods Research

Criteria to score separately the methodological quality of the qualitative and quantitative strands of a study:
- Criteria for scoring the qualitative strand of the study
- Criteria for scoring the quantitative strand of the study

Criteria that are explicitly concerned with mixed methods research:
- Mixing and integration of methods
- Rationale for mixing methods stated

Generic critical appraisal criteria:
- Design
- Interpretation, conclusions, inferences, and implications
- Data analysis
- Research aims and questions
- Sampling and data collection
- Theoretical framework
- Impact of investigator
- Transparency
- Context

From Heyvaert, M., Hannes, K., Maes, B., Onghena, P. 2013. Critical appraisal of mixed methods studies. J. Mixed Methods Res. 7 (4), 302–327.

Thus we recommend that the qualitative and quantitative components of mixed methods studies should be appraised against the criteria described in Chapters 4 and 5, and as well as the additional criteria that are explicitly concerned with MMR (Table 6.2) and are discussed in the following sections.

REPORTING MIXED METHODS RESEARCH

In 2008, O'Cathain published guidelines for reporting MMR: Good reporting of Mixed Methods Studies (GRAMMS, Box 6.3) (O'Cathain et al., 2008). In addition to criteria relating to study design and methods, O'Cathain et al. also included criteria requiring that the personnel involved in integration should be reported, together with a description of their insights gained from the integration, in a similar way that reflexivity is a component of reporting in qualitative studies.

Some individual journals also provide specific guidelines for reporting MMR, but this is not widespread, and the detail provided to guide authors varies considerably (e.g., see the *Journal of Mixed Methods Research, Journal of Advanced Nursing,* and *Global Qualitative Nursing Research*).

Applying Mixed Methods Research to Practice

All research starts with formulating an answerable question and then designing a study using the most appropriate method. We hope that this chapter, and the many examples within it, has helped you to better understand the use of MMR as a method, especially evident in complex health care and health promotion. The next stage in this process is for you to consider how MMR is applied to your own practice and how you can influence change by basing your practice on the best available evidence. To do this, we have given you a scenario. See Box 6.4. We suggest that you appraise it using the criteria in Table 6.2. A model answer can be found in Table 6.3.

TABLE 6.2 ■ **Criteria for Appraising Mixed Methods Studies**

	Criteria	Response	Reason for Response/ Comment
Design			
1	Is there a description of the philosophy or theory informing the research and the ways this philosophy or theory shapes the investigation?		
2	Did the study ask a clearly focused research question?		
3	Is there a rationale for why a mixed methods study design is needed to address the research question?		
4	Does the study use a convergent parallel, explanatory sequential, exploratory sequential, or other defined mixed method? Is the chosen mixed methods study design appropriate to address the study aims?		
Conduct			
5	What was the overall judgment of the qualitative study quality?		
6	What was the overall judgment of the quantitative study quality?		
7	Is there a clear description of where integration occurs (either at study design level, methods level, and/or interpretation level)?		
8	If integration occurs at the methods level (sampling, data collection, data analysis), are the methods clearly described?		
Analysis			
9	If integration occurs at the data interpretation and reporting stage, are the methods clearly described, and are meta-inferences based on the interpretation of data from the component studies?		
Overall Judgment			
10	What is the overall judgment of the value of this mixed methods study? Can the results be applied in your context?		

BOX 6.3 ■ **O'Cathain's Good Reporting of Mixed Methods Studies (GRAMMS)**

- Describe the justification for using a mixed methods approach to the research question.
- Describe the design in terms of the purpose, priority, and sequence of methods.
- Describe each method in terms of sampling, data collection, and analysis.
- Describe where integration has occurred, how it has occurred, and who has participated in it.
- Describe any limitation of one method associated with the presence of the other method.
- Describe any insights gained from mixing or integrating methods.

From O'Cathain, A., Murphy, E., Nicholl, J., 2008. The quality of mixed methods studies in health services research. J. Health Serv. Res. Policy 13 (2), 92–98.

BOX 6.4 ■ Example of a Scenario to Develop a Support Program for Nurses Experiencing Stress in Neonatal Intensive Care Units

Scenario

You are a nurse manager and are concerned about the health of the nurses in your team due to the stressful situations that they encounter when looking after acutely ill babies.

Evidence

Beck, C.T., Cusson, R.M., et al., 2017. Secondary traumatic stress in NICU nurses. Adv. Neonatal Care 17 (6), 478–488.

Aim of the Study

The study had two aims. Firstly, to determine the prevalence and severity of traumatic stress in neonatal intensive care units (NICU) (using quantitative methods) and secondly to explore nurses experiences (using qualitative methods).

Results Reported in the Study

The quantitative findings found that nurses experience moderate to severe secondary traumatic stress. The qualitative findings found five major themes: (1) "What Intensified NICU Nurses' Traumatic Experiences"; (2) "Parents Insisting on Aggressive Treatment"; (3) "Baby Torture: Performing Painful Procedures"; (4) "Questioning Their Skills: Did I Do Enough?"; and (5) "The Grief of the Family: It Is Contagious."

My Summary Appraisal of the Paper and its Application to My Practice

By using mixed methods, this study has quantified the extent of the problem of secondary stress in NICU staff and enhanced these findings by using qualitative methods to illustrate the effects this has on staff. This study appears to fit in with the context of my own working environment, although I have some cautions regarding the results due to the very low response rate.

This paper has provided useful evidence for me to present to my managers a plan to develop a support program for the nurses in my own NICU unit, for example, in recognizing the signs of secondary traumatic stress and assistance that is needed to support our nurses in the longer term.

TABLE 6.3 ■ Assessing the Quality of a Study Investigating the Prevalence and Severity of Traumatic Stress Among Nurses Working in Neonatal Intensive Care Units. A Worked Example Using Quality Criteria Described In Table 6.2

	Criteria	Response	Reason for Response/Comment
Design			
1	Is there a description of the philosophy or theory informing the research and the ways this philosophy or theory shapes the investigation?	Yes	The authors state that pragmatism was the paradigm that underpinned the study.
2	Did the study ask a clearly focused research question?	Yes	A summary literature review is included in this paper, which has informed the research. There are three research questions. (1) To determine the prevalence and severity of secondary traumatic stress in neonatal intensive care units (NICUs) (using quantitative methods); (2) to explore nurses experiences (using qualitative methods); and (3) to use the results from (1) and (2) to develop a more complete picture.

Table 6.3 ■ Assessing the Quality of a Study Investigating the Prevalence and Severity of Traumatic Stress Among Nurses Working in Neonatal Intensive Care Units. A Worked Example Using Quality Criteria Described In Table 6.2—cont'd

	Criteria	Response	Reason for Response/Comment
3	Is there a rationale for why a mixed methods study design is needed to address the research question?	Yes	The authors clearly state that by using mixed methods they are aiming to develop a more complete understanding. They also state that the quantitative and qualitative strands had equal weight.
4	Does the study use a convergent parallel, explanatory sequential, exploratory sequential, or other defined mixed method? Is the chosen mixed methods study design appropriate to address the study aims?	Yes	The authors clearly state that they used a convergent parallel design, and this is illustrated in Figure 6.1. in the paper. This appears to be an appropriate design as the authors conducted the quantitative and qualitative studies in parallel, with equal priority given to both strands, and integration occurred at the interpretation stage. This design addresses the study aims appropriately.
Conduct			
5	What is the overall judgment of the qualitative study quality?	See comments box	62% of respondents completed the qualitative section, and their free text ranged from one paragraph to two full pages of typed text. Data do not appear to have been independently coded. Two authors agreed the five themes. Quotes used to support themes within text and in Figure 6.3 in the paper. Tables 6.3 and 6.4 in the paper give examples of helpful and unhelpful practices.
6	What is the overall judgment of the quantitative study quality?	See comments box	There was a very low response rate to the survey (3%). Respondents were mainly staff nurses and white women. Experience of working as a NICU nurse ranged from 1–43 years. Informative descriptive statistics table.
7	Is there a clear description of where integration occurs (either at study design level, methods level, and/or interpretation level)?	Yes	At the methods and data interpretation stages; for details, see next questions.
8	If integration occurs at the methods level (sampling, data collection, data analysis), are the methods clearly described?	Yes	The sample consisted of NICU nurses. Data were collected via an electronic survey that used a validated tool to collect quantitative data and a free text section where participants were asked to describe their experiences. Quantitative data were analyzed using descriptive statistics and content analysis used for the qualitative data.

Continued

Table 6.3 ■ Assessing the Quality of a Study Investigating the Prevalence and Severity of Traumatic Stress Among Nurses Working in Neonatal Intensive Care Units. A Worked Example Using Quality Criteria Described In Table 6.2—cont'd

	Criteria	Response	Reason for Response/Comment
Analysis			
9	If integration occurs at the data interpretation and reporting stage, are the methods clearly described, and have meta-inferences been based on the interpretation of data from the component studies?	Yes	Quantitative and qualitative data were merged by presenting qualitative quotes alongside the quantitative findings and also by using side-by-side comparison to compare the results from the different data. The study is illustrated in a flow diagram (see Figure 6.1) demonstrating that data were collected in parallel and then merged after data collection.
Overall Judgment			
10	What is the overall judgment of the value of this mixed methods study? Can the results be applied in your context?	See comments box	By using mixed methods, this study has quantified the extent of the problem of secondary stress in NICU staff and enhanced these findings by using qualitative methods to illustrate the effects this has on them. This study appears to fit in with the context of my own working environment, although I have some cautions regarding the results due to the very low response rate.
			This paper has given me useful evidence for me to present to my managers to develop a support program for the nurses in my own NICU unit (e.g., in recognizing signs of secondary traumatic stress and assistance that is needed to support our nurses in the longer term).

Summary

In this chapter, we have explained how the emerging methodology of MMR encompasses both quantitative and qualitative methods in a single study, or program of inquiry. We have shown that it is much more than simply collecting both qualitative and quantitative data and combining the findings. MMR aims to provide a better understanding of complex phenomena. As health care is progressively complex, mixed methods are ideally suited to work with this complexity. In addition to explaining the premise and processes inherent in conducting MMR, this chapter has also given you guidance in critically appraising it. As MMR is increasingly being used by nurse researchers to develop evidence-based care and inform clinical nursing practice, there is a need for nurses to be aware of the skills needed to assess the quality of MMR before deciding on its application to practice. We hope this chapter has helped you to start on this journey.

Exercise

We encourage you to consolidate your learning by visiting our companion website to access a scenario relevant to nursing practice, which has a blank template for you to complete and a model answer.

References

Ankuda, C.K., et al., 2018. What matters most? A mixed methods study of critical aspects of a home-based palliative program. Am. J. Hosp. Palliative Care 35 (2), 236–243.

Beck, C.T., et al., 2017. Secondary traumatic stress in NICU nurses: a mixed-methods study. Adv. Neonatal Care 17 (6), 478–488.

Beck, C.T., Harrison, L., 2016. Mixed-methods research in the discipline of nursing. Adv. Nurs. Sci. 39 (3), 224–234.

Bryman, A., 2007. Barriers to integrating quantitative and qualitative research. J. Mixed Methods Res. 1 (1), 8–22.

Burke Johnson, R., Onwuegbuzie, A., 2004. Mixed methods research: a research paradigm whose time has come. Educ. Res. 33 (7), 14–26.

Burke Johnson, R., Onwuegbuzie, A., Turner, L., 2007. Toward a definition of mixed methods research. J. Mixed Methods Res. 1 (2), 112–133.

Centers for Disease Control and Prevention, 2008. Introduction to Process Evaluation in Tobacco Use Prevention and Control. Atlanta. Available from: https://www.cdc.gov/tobacco/stateandcommunity/tobacco_control_programs/surveillance_evaluation/process_evaluation/index.htm (accessed 22.2.18).

Creswell, J., 2015. A Concise Introduction to Mixed Methods Research. Sage Publications, London.

Creswell, J.W., et al., 2011. Best Practices for Mixed Methods Research in the Health Sciences. Office of Behavioral and Social Sciences Research, National Institutes of Health, Washington, D.C.

Dane, A.V., Schneider, B.H., 1998. Program integrity in primary and early secondary prevention: are implementation effects out of control? Clin. Psychol. Rev. 18 (1), 23–45.

Desborough, J., et al., 2018. Developing a positive patient experience with nurses in general practice: an integrated model of patient satisfaction and enablement. J. Adv. Nurs. 74 (3), 564–578. Available from: http://doi.wiley.com/10.1111/jan.13461.

Fàbregues, S., Molina-Azorín, J.F., 2017. Addressing quality in mixed methods research: a review and recommendations for a future agenda. Qual. Quant. 51 (6), 2847–2863. Available from: http://link.springer.com/10.1007/s11135-016-0449-4 (accessed 6.5.19).

Farquhar, M.C., Ewing, G., Booth, S., 2011. Using mixed methods to develop and evaluate complex interventions in palliative care research. Palliat. Med. 25 (8), 748–757.

Fetters, M.D., Curry, L.A., Creswell, J.W., 2013. Achieving integration in mixed methods designs—principles and practices. Health Serv. Res. 48 (6 Part 2), 2134–2156.

Fetters, M.D., Molina-Azorín, J.F., 2017. The Journal of Mixed Methods Research starts a new decade: the mixed methods research integration trilogy and its dimensions. J. Mixed Methods Res. 11 (3), 291–307.

Greenwood, N., Habibi, R., 2014. Carer mentoring: a mixed methods investigation of a carer mentoring service. Int. J. Nurs. Stud. 51 (3), 359–369. Available from: https://doi.org/10.1016/j.ijnurstu.2013.06.011.

Guise, J.M., et al., 2017. AHRQ series on complex intervention systematic reviews—paper 1: an introduction to a series of articles that provide guidance and tools for reviews of complex interventions. J. Clin. Epidemiol. 90, 6–10. Available from: https://doi.org/10.1016/j.jclinepi.2017.06.011>.

Hanson, S., Cross, J., Jones, A., 2016. Promoting physical activity interventions in communities with poor health and socio-economic profiles: a process evaluation of the implementation of a new walking group scheme. Soc. Sci. Med. 169, 77–85. Available from: https://doi.org/10.1016/j.socscimed.2016.09.035.

Heyvaert, M., et al., 2013. Critical appraisal of mixed methods studies. J. Mixed Methods Res. 7 (4), 302–327.

Marino, C., Child, B., Krasinski, V.C., 2016. Sharing Experience Learned Firsthand (SELF): self-disclosure of lived experience in mental health services and supports. Psychiatr. Rehabil. J. 39 (2), 154–160.

Mason, J., 2006. Mixing methods in a qualitatively driven way. Qual. Res. 6 (1), 9–25.

Moffatt, S., et al., 2006. Using quantitative and qualitative data in health services research—What happens when mixed method findings conflict? [ISRCTN61522618]. BMC Health Serv. Res. 6, 1–10.

O'Cathain, A., Murphy, E., Nicholl, J., 2008. The quality of mixed methods studies in health services research. J. Health Serv. Res. Policy 13 (2), 92–98.

O'Cathain, A., et al., 2013. What can qualitative research do for randomised controlled trials? A systematic mapping review. BMJ Open 3 (6), BMJ Open 2013;3:e002889. https://doi.org/10.1136/bmjopen-2013-002889.

O'Cathain, A., Murphy, E., Nicholl, J., 2010. Three techniques for integrating data in mixed methods studies. BMJ 341, c4587.

Onwuegbuzie, A.J., et al., 2007. Conducting mixed analyses: a general typology. Int. J. Mult. Res. Approaches 1 (1), 4–17.

Ozawa, S., Pongpirul, K., 2014. 10 Best Resources on.. mixed methods research in health systems. Health Policy Planning 29 (3), 323–327.

Plano Clark, V., 2010. The adoption and practice of mixed methods: U.S. trends in federally funded health-related research. Qual. Inq. 16, 428–440.

Pluye, P., Hong, Q.N., 2014. Combining the power of stories and the power of numbers: mixed methods research and mixed studies reviews. Ann. Rev. Public Health 35 (1), 29–45.

Sackett, D., et al., 2000. Evidence-Based Medicine: How to Practice and Teach EBM, second ed. Churchill Livingstone, Edinburgh.

Schifferdecker, K.E., Reed, V., 2009. Using mixed methods research in medical education: basic guidelines for researchers. Med. Educ. 43, 637–644.

Shorten, A., Smith, J., 2017. Mixed methods research: expanding the evidence base. Evid. Based Nurs. 20 (3), 74.

Steckler, A., Linnan, L., 2002. Process Evaluation for Public Health Interventions and Research. Jossey Bass, San Francisco, CA.

U.S. Government Accountability Office, 2011. Performance Measurement and Evaluation: Definition and Relationships. Available from: https://www.gao.gov/new.items/d11646sp.pdf (accessed 6.5.19).

Weldam, S.W., et al., 2017. Nurses' perspectives of a new individualized nursing care intervention for COPD patients in primary care settings: a mixed method study. Appl. Nurs. Res. 33, 85–92. Available from: https://doi.org/10.1016/j.apnr.2016.10.010.

Further Reading

Brannen, J., 2009. Prologue mixed methods for novice researchers: reflections and themes. Int. J. Mult. Res. Approaches 3 (1), 8–12.

Bryman, A., 2007. Barriers to integrating quantitative and qualitative research. J. Mixed Methods Res. 1 (1), 8–22.

Bryman, A., 2006. Editorial. Qualitative research, 6. Sage Publications, Thousand Oaks, CA, pp. 5–7 (1). Available from: http://qrj.sagepub.com/cgi/doi/10.1177/1468794106058865 (accessed 22.2.18).

Burke Johnson, R., Onwuegbuzie, A., Turner, L., 2007. Toward a definition of mixed methods research. J. Mixed Methods Res. 1 (2), 112–133.

O'Cathain, A., Murphy, E., Nicholl, J., 2008. The quality of mixed methods studies in health services research. J. Health Serv. Res. Policy 13 (2), 92–98.

Creswell, J., 2015. A Concise Introduction to Mixed Methods Research. Sage Publications, London.

Creswell, J., Plano Clark, V., 2011. Designing and Conducting Mixed Methods Research, second ed. Sage Publications, Thousand Oaks, CA.

Creswell, J., Plano Clark, V., 2018. Designing and Conducting Mixed Methods Research, third ed. Sage Publications, Thousand Oaks, CA.

Farquhar, M.C., Ewing, G., Booth, S., 2011. Using mixed methods to develop and evaluate complex interventions in palliative care research. Palliat. Med. 25 (8), 748–757.

Fetters, M.D., Curry, L.A., Creswell, J.W., 2013. Achieving integration in mixed methods designs—principles and practices. Health Serv. Res. 48 (6 Part 2), 2134–2156.

Green, J., 2007. Mixed Methods in Social Inquiry. John Wiley & Sons, San Francisco, CA.

Mason, J., 2006. Mixing methods in a qualitatively driven way. Qual. Res. 6 (1), 9–25.

Morgan, D.L., 2007. Paradigms lost and pragmatism regained: methodological implications of combining qualitative and quantitative methods. Mixed Methods Res. 1 (1), 48–76.

Onwuegbuzie, A., Burke Johnson, R., 2006. The validity issue in mixed research. Res. Schools 13 (1), 48–63.

Onwuegbuzie, A., Leech, N., 2005. On becoming a pragmatic researcher: the importance of combining quantitative and qualitative research methodologies. Int. J. Soc. Res. Method. 8 (5), 375–387.

Plano Clark, V., Ivankova, N., 2016. Mixed Methods Research: A Guide to the Field, third ed. Sage Publications, Thousand Oaks, CA.

Sale, J., Brazil, K., 2004. A strategy to identify critical appraisal criteria for primary mixed-method studies. Qual. Quant. 38 (4), 351–365.

Tashakkori, A., Teddlie, C., 2010. Handbook of Mixed Methods in Social and Behavioral Research, second ed. Sage Publications, Thousand Oaks, CA.

CHAPTER 7

Using Evidence from Systematic Reviews

Kate Flemming ■ Leanne V. Jones

KEY POINTS

- Systematic reviews use rigorous methods to reduce bias and can provide reliable summaries of research evidence.
- Because systematic reviews include a comprehensive search, appraisal, and synthesis of research evidence, they can provide shortcuts in the evidence-based process.
- The Cochrane Library, which is updated regularly and available online, includes a database of up-to-date systematic reviews from across the whole of health care.
- PROSPERO, available online and regularly updated, includes registered protocols (research proposals) for systematic reviews in health, social care, welfare, public health, education, crime, justice, and international development.
- Critical appraisal of systematic reviews is necessary to ensure that they have met quality standards.
- Systematic reviews can summarize research evidence from quantitative (randomized controlled trials [RCTs], cohort studies, case-control studies) or qualitative research, or can integrate both qualitative and quantitative research evidence.
- Systematic reviews of quantitative study designs (e.g., RCTs) may include meta-analyses. A meta-analysis is a statistical technique used to combine data from multiple studies, to answer the questions "does this intervention have a beneficial effect?" and if so, "what is the size of that effect?"
- There are various methods for systematic reviews of qualitative research including thematic synthesis, framework synthesis, and meta-ethnography.

What are Systematic Reviews?

Reviews of healthcare literature take many forms depending on the audience to which they are addressed. They may include chapters in textbooks, reports to expert committees, and "state-of-the-art" reviews for clinical journals. The main purpose of these reviews is to bring their audience rapidly up to speed with the current information in specific clinical areas.

Healthcare professionals at every stage of their career development often feel overwhelmed by the magnitude of literature available to them, and have increasingly come to rely on summaries of the evidence in the form of reviews. Many of these review articles are well researched, beautifully illustrated, and highly entertaining and informative. However, as "bottom-line" summaries of which treatments, diagnostic tests, and so on, are effective, they can be misleading. One reason for this is that reviews are often written by acknowledged experts, who are likely to have already formed an opinion about what works, and who may not review the evidence in an unbiased manner. Another reason is that writing reviews is not always regarded as the most important academic activity, and less time is devoted to it than, for example, writing original research. So those writing the reviews may cut corners and rehash something they have written previously, rather than undertaking an exhaustive search for and critical appraisal of all the evidence.

Let us take the example quoted by Professor Paul Knipschild in the seminal book *Systematic Reviews* (Knipschild, 1995). He describes how the distinguished biochemist Linus Pauling, writing in his book *How to Live Long and Feel Better* (Pauling, 1986), quoted more than 30 trials that supported his contention that vitamin C could prevent the common cold. Knipschild et al. then went on to do their own "systematic review," which showed that even large doses of vitamin C cannot prevent a cold, although they may slightly decrease its duration and severity. A critical review of what Pauling had written showed that he had omitted a number of important studies that did not support the contention that he so enthusiastically proposed. There are now many examples that have shown that unsystematic reviews (defined here as "literature reviews") do not routinely incorporate all relevant up-to-date scientific evidence.

This shortcoming has led to the notion that reviews need to be performed systematically. This means that the same rigor that we expect of people undertaking primary research should be demanded of reviewers undertaking this very important task of "research synthesis" or "secondary research." You have seen from Chapter 5 that in studies such as RCTs, the study can be designed so that bias is reduced, one example being the use of blinding (or masking) investigators, participants, and interventionists as to whether participants are in the experimental or the control group. In the same way, strategies can be introduced to the reviewing process to reduce the human element of bias caused, for example, by the reviewer having a strong opinion about whether the treatment under review works.

The steps in the systematic review process are outlined in Box 7.1. In the first part of this chapter we focus on systematic reviews of quantitative research. We then discuss systematic reviews of qualitative research.

SYSTEMATIC REVIEWS OF QUANTITATIVE RESEARCH
Developing a Protocol

A systematic review protocol is written before the systematic review starts. It outlines the rationale for the systematic review, the question(s) to be addressed, and the methods to be used. Publication of

---

BOX 7.1 ■ How to Conduct a Systematic Review

1. Develop a protocol outlining the rationale for the systematic review, the review question(s), and the detailed methods for the review.
2. Ensure that the review question(s) is clearly defined.
3. Ensure that there are clear inclusion and exclusion criteria to guide which types of studies are eligible for inclusion in the systematic review.
4. Perform a comprehensive search of all relevant sources for potentially eligible studies.
5. Examine the studies to decide eligibility (if possible with two independent reviewers).
6. Construct a table describing the characteristics of the included studies.
7. Assess methodological quality of included studies (if possible with two independent reviewers).
8. Extract data (with a second investigator if possible) with involvement of other investigators if necessary.
9. Analyze and synthesize results of included studies using statistical synthesis (meta-analysis) if appropriate, or a narrative synthesis.
10. Prepare a report of review summarizing methods and any deviations from protocol, and describing results and conclusions.

a protocol of a review before knowledge of the available studies reduces the impact of review authors' biases, promotes transparency of methods and processes, allows peer review of the planned methods, and reduces the potential for duplication (Green and Higgins, 2011). Protocols can be prospectively registered in PROSPERO, an international database of systematic reviews in health and social care, welfare, public health, education, crime, justice, and international development. Prospectively publishing a protocol is what largely distinguishes a systematic review from a literature review.

The Research Question

Systematic reviews can address a wide range of questions from determining the effectiveness of an intervention, to the prognosis of a condition, to the accuracy of a diagnostic test. The reviewer needs to define his or her question(s) very precisely as the entire methods for the systematic review flow from the question(s).

Inclusion and Exclusion Criteria

An explicit list of eligibility criteria is needed. This guides the reviewers when they are selecting studies to include in the review, thereby reducing the risk of study selection bias.

To illustrate, here are the clearly defined eligibility criteria published by Francis et al. in their systematic review entitled "Oral protein calorie supplementation for children with chronic disease" (Francis et al., 2015). Studies were eligible if participants were children 1 to 16 years of age with any disease that requires medical intervention for a period of 6 months or more; interventions were oral protein calorie supplements of any amount given for at least 1 month; comparisons were routine nutritional advice or placebo or no intervention; outcomes were change in nutritional indices or one or more of other outcomes (they listed these); study designs were randomized and quasi-randomized controlled trials.

Searching for Literature and What to Include

The search should be thorough including electronic databases (e.g., MEDLINE) and also, where possible, sources of unpublished studies. This may seem odd, but there is a phenomenon known as "publication bias": for any intervention, there may be studies that do not show a clear benefit of the intervention, and these studies are less likely to be published (Dwan et al., 2013). Excluding unpublished studies from systematic reviews may bias the results of the review toward studies in which a benefit of the intervention was observed. One approach to identifying unpublished studies is to search for abstracts of studies presented at conferences, available in the abstract books of relevant international conferences.

Depending on the topic under investigation, the search may need to be designed to identify both English and non-English language articles. An example is in the field of complementary medicine; many studies of acupuncture may be published in non-English language journals, particularly those from China (Ma et al., 2016).

Study Selection

Once the search has been conducted, the next step is to select eligible studies using the pre-determined inclusion and exclusion criteria. To reduce bias in study selection, it is best if more than one reviewer does this, and that they work independently of one another. The reviewers can then compare which studies they have independently included. They should have previously agreed on a mechanism for resolving any differences between their lists of included studies. This may mean involving a third reviewer.

Constructing a Table of Characteristics

The next step is to tabulate the characteristics (methods, details of the participants, the precise nature of the interventions, and the outcomes measured) of the included studies. By tabulating the characteristics of all studies that have been identified as eligible by one or more reviewers, it will soon become apparent whether the inclusion criteria really have been fulfilled. The final table of included studies, which all reviewers have agreed, will appear in the review, and the readers can judge if the reviewers got it right. For each study excluded at this point, the reviewers need to state, in the review, the reason for this exclusion, and again the reader can judge whether this is valid.

When reading a review, examination of the "characteristics of included studies" can help the reader decide whether the review is applicable to his or her question. The reader may want evidence for a specific age group. If none of the studies has included this age group, then they will need to carefully consider whether the review findings are relevant for their needs.

In addition to the data extracted to the "characteristics of included studies" table, other important data such as the results (see the "Data Synthesis" section later in this chapter) and key methodological features should be extracted from each study.

Assessing Risk of Bias and Quality of the Evidence

The next step in the review process is to assess the methodological quality (risk of bias) of the included studies. Again, it is best if these steps are performed by more than one person, using an appropriate checklist. There are many checklists now available. In Cochrane systematic reviews, each study is assessed to judge whether it has a low, high, or unclear risk of bias (Higgins et al., 2011). Studies deemed at high risk of bias are either excluded (this would need to have been decided at the outset and stated in the protocol), or alternatively, included but analyzed separately from studies deemed at low risk of bias. In a systematic review examining the effects of support for healthy breastfeeding mothers (McFadden et al., 2017), a pooled analysis of all studies indicated that breastfeeding mothers who had support were more likely to still be breastfeeding up to 6 months postbirth. A separate analysis, retaining only those studies at low risk of bias, again indicated a positive effect of support on breastfeeding. This analysis, known as a "sensitivity analysis," provided reassurance that the overall pooled results were not affected by including the higher risk of bias studies.

In addition to assessing the risk of bias of included studies, it is now mandatory in Cochrane reviews to assess the quality of the whole body of evidence for each important outcome according to five factors: study limitations (risk of bias), consistency of effect (heterogeneity), imprecision, indirectness, and publication bias. This is known as the GRADE (Grading of Recommendations, Assessment, Development, and Evaluation) approach (Schünemann et al., 2013). GRADE assessments are done once all meta-analyses have been completed. The "intervention effect" and a measure of quality for each key outcome is summarized in a "Summary of Findings" table. The quality of evidence for each outcome across all the studies is then assessed against the five factors, and can be downgraded depending on the outcome of the assessments.

Data Synthesis

The next step in the review process is to synthesize the extracted data, either statistically or narratively. The methods for data synthesis should be defined clearly in advance within the protocol.

The effect of an intervention can be measured in various ways. For instance, there may be various measures of nutritional status, as there were in the review by Francis et al. on oral protein calorie supplementation (Francis et al., 2015). Nutritional status could be ascertained by taking measures of weight and height. These measures are known as "continuous": the data can take any value in a specified range. There may also be "dichotomous" (binary) outcome data: the outcome for every participant is one of two possibilities, for example, dead or alive, or clinical improvement or no clinical improvement. In a systematic review, if all the clinical trials are measuring the same outcome measures in the same way, then it may be appropriate to statistically combine the data in a meta-analysis. The summary statistics commonly used for meta-analysis of continuous data are the mean difference (MD) and the standardized mean difference (SMD), and for meta-analysis

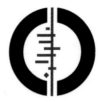

Fig. 7.1 The Cochrane Collaboration logo, indicating a meta-analysis of seven randomized controlled trials comparing corticosteroids versus no corticosteroids in pregnant women about to deliver prematurely. (Copyright Cochrane Collaboration, reproduced with permission. Available from: http://www.cochrane.org.)

of dichotomous data are the risk ratio (RR) and the odds ratio (OR) (Deeks et al., 2011). In some situations, statistical analysis of the results may not be possible or appropriate. For example, slightly different measurements of outcomes may have been made in each of the included trials, so they cannot be combined as one summary outcome measure. This is referred to as "heterogeneity" (explained more fully later in this chapter). In this situation, reviewers should summarize the results of individual studies, in narrative or tabular form.

Understanding Meta-analysis

Statistical synthesis involves combining the data from the included studies in a process referred to as "meta-analysis." It can be very powerful. The individual studies that make up a review are, on their own, often small and unable to detect whether or not a treatment is effective, but when the data from a number of similar small studies are combined, valid conclusions may be drawn. Often the terms "meta-analysis" and "systematic review" are used interchangeably. This is inappropriate because, as can be seen from Box 7.1, meta-analysis is simply one of the final steps in a systematic review. It provides no reassurance that the individual studies included in the meta-analysis were reviewed systematically or appropriately. The most important steps in a systematic review are those that we have already described, which are set up to prevent bias.

The Cochrane logo (Fig. 7.1) is a stylized diagram of a meta-analysis from a systematic review that included data from seven RCTs, which investigated the effect of corticosteroids administered to pregnant women who were about to deliver prematurely. The outcome examined was the survival of their infant. The vertical line is where these results would be expected to cluster if this treatment had a similar effect to the control group (placebo or no treatment) and each horizontal line represents the results of one trial. The shorter the line, the more certain the result, because the 95% confidence intervals are narrow. If the horizontal line lies entirely to the left of the vertical line, the treatment has shown significant benefit. If it touches or crosses the vertical line, then clear benefit was not demonstrated in that trial. If the horizontal line were to lie entirely to the right of the vertical line, then more babies would have died in the treatment group than in the control group, that is, the treatment would have been harmful. The trial at the top of the diagram was performed in 1972 and did show benefit, but the four subsequent trials did not. The sixth trial did show benefit, and the seventh did not. On a simple "vote count" (five of the trials showed no benefit), one might be persuaded not to use this intervention. However, when a systematic review was performed with meta-analysis and first reported in 1989 (Crowley 1996), this showed that corticosteroids administered to pregnant women reduced the odds of their babies dying by between 30% and 50%. This pooled result is indicated by the solid diamond at the bottom of the diagram.

Meta-analysis can answer two main questions about a treatment: "Does this intervention have a beneficial (or harmful) effect?" and if so "What is the size of that effect?" First, we will explain some terms used in expressing results, starting with "relative risk" (or risk ratio). The risk (or proportion, probability, or rate) is the ratio of people with an event in a group compared with the total in that group. In Table 7.1, the risk of the outcome being present in group 1 is:

TABLE 7.1 ■ How Results of a Prospective Study Are Represented

		Group 1	Group 2	Total
Outcome present	Yes	a	b	a + b
	No	c	d	c + d
	Total	a + c	b + d	n

TABLE 7.2 ■ Relation Between Epidural Use and Self-Hypnosis for Pain Management in Labor

		Self-Hypnosis	Usual Care	Total
Using epidural analgesia	Yes	a	b	a + b
during labor		112	132	244
	No	c	d	c + d
		225	198	423
	Total	a + c	b + d	n
		337	330	667

Data from Downe, S., Finlayson, K., Melvin, C., Spiby, H., Ali, S., Diggle, P., et al., 2015. Self-hypnosis for intra-partum pain management in pregnant nulliparous women: a randomised controlled trial of clinical effective-ness. BJOG 122 (9), 1226–1234. https://doi.org/%2010.1111/1471-0528.13433.

$$a/(a+c)$$

In 2015, a clinical trial published by Downe et al. (2015) compared self-hypnosis with usual care for pain management in pregnant women during labor. The outcome that we will consider is use of epidural analgesia for labor pain relief. There were 337 women in the self-hypnosis group and 330 women in the usual care group. Table 7.2 shows the numbers in each group who used epidural analgesia. So the risk of using epidural analgesia is 112/337 in the self-hypnosis group and 132/330 in the usual care group.

The relative risk is the ratio of the risk in the intervention group to the risk in the control group. For this trial, the relative risk is:

$$\frac{112/337}{132/330} = \frac{0.33}{0.40} = 0.83$$

If the risk in the treatment and the comparison groups is the same, the ratio will be 1. Here the ratio is less than 1 (0.83), which means the risk of using epidural anesthesia is lower in the self-hypnosis group compared with the usual care group.

The "odds ratio" is the ratio of the odds of an event in the treatment group compared with the odds of an event in the comparison group. The odds are the ratio of the number of people in a group with an event compared with the number without an event. So, looking again at Table 7.1, the odds of a patient in group 1 having the outcome present are:

$$a/c$$

In the Downe trial, the odds of using epidural analgesia in the self-hypnosis group are:

$$112/225 = 0.50$$

In the usual care group, the odds of using epidural analgesia are:

$$132/198 = 0.67$$

The odds ratio of using epidural analgesia for labor pain relief in the two groups is:

TABLE 7.3 ■ Midwife-Led Continuity Models Versus Other Models of Care for Childbearing Women*

Study or Subgroup	Midwife-led care Events	Total	Other models of care Events	Total	Weight	Risk Ratio M-H, Random, 95% CI	Risk Ratio M-H, Random, 95% CI
Begley 2011	139	1096	79	549	8.8%	0.88 [0.68, 1.14]	
Biro 2000	67	488	86	480	6.7%	0.77 [0.57, 1.03]	
Flint 1989	56	503	66	498	5.2%	0.84 [0.60, 1.17]	
Harvey 1996	6	105	7	97	0.5%	0.79 [0.28, 2.27]	
Homer 2001	71	593	63	601	5.7%	1.14 [0.83, 1.57]	
Kenny 1994	12	194	29	211	1.4%	0.45 [0.24, 0.86]	
MacVicar 1993	187	2304	114	1206	11.7%	0.86 [0.69, 1.07]	
McLachlan 2012	202	1150	222	1157	19.5%	0.92 [0.77, 1.09]	
North Stafford 2000	74	770	84	735	6.6%	0.84 [0.63, 1.13]	
Rowley 1995	29	405	37	409	2.7%	0.79 [0.50, 1.26]	
Tracy 2013	172	851	171	841	16.2%	0.99 [0.82, 1.20]	
Turnbull 1996	83	643	86	635	7.3%	0.95 [0.72, 1.26]	
Waldenstrorm 2001	78	484	89	496	7.6%	0.90 [0.68, 1.18]	
Total (95% CI)		9586		7915	100.0%	0.90 [0.83, 0.97]	
Total events	1176		1133				

Heterogeneity: Tau^2 = 0.00; Chi^2 = 9.91, df = 12 (P = 0.62); I^2 = 0%
Test for overall effect: Z = 2.79 (P = 0.005)

0.1 0.2 0.5 1 2 5 10
Favors midwifery Favors other models

*The outcome is instrumental vaginal birth (RR and 95% Confidence Interval).
Copyright Cochrane Library, with permission.

$$0.50/0.67 = 0.75$$

If the odds of the event in the treatment and the comparison groups are the same, then the odds ratio is again 1. That is, there is no difference between the treatment and comparison groups. Again, the odds ratio indicates that women in the self-hypnosis group were less likely than those in the usual care group to use epidural analgesia for labor pain relief.

Where the outcome of interest is rare, in Table 7.1, a will be very small and $a/(a + c)$ will be approximately equal to a/c. Similarly, $b/(b + d)$ will approximately equal b/d. Thus, when the outcome is rare, the risks of the outcomes in the two groups will be very similar to the odds of the outcomes in the two groups, and the relative risks will be very similar to the odds ratios.

Ninety-five percent confidence intervals are an expression of how precise the estimate of the odds ratio or relative risk is. This gives an estimate of the range to 95% certainty that the true result for odds ratio or relative risk lies within the range stated.

Let us consider now a systematic review by Sandall et al., which compared the effects of midwife-led continuity models of care with other models of care for childbearing women and their infants (Sandall et al., 2016). The review included 15 trials randomizing a total of 17,674 women to either midwife-led continuity models of care or other models of care during pregnancy and birth. One of the outcomes investigated was instrumental vaginal birth (forceps or ventouse). Thirteen trials reported on this outcome. This meta-analysis is illustrated in Table 7.3. The ratios shown in the column labeled "Midwife-led care" indicate the number of patients in the experimental group who had an instrumental vaginal birth compared with the total number of patients in that group. These risks are shown both for each individual study and, at the bottom, for the thirteen studies combined.

Now look at the final column. You will see a number of "blobs" bisected by horizontal lines. Reading the figures along the bottom axis, the position of the blob represents the risk ratio for each individual trial. The horizontal line represents the 95% confidence interval of the individual trial. In this situation, if both the risk ratio and the 95% confidence interval lie entirely to the left of the vertical line at 1, it means there is a statistically significant benefit, in this case of midwife-led models compared with other models of care, for the outcome being examined (instrumental vaginal birth). If one looks at the 13 individual trials, it will be seen that this applies to only one trial (Kenny). In the other trials, the horizontal line crosses the vertical line of 1. This means that, although the risk ratio lies to the left of the line for some trials such as Biro, the 95% confidence intervals include the line of no effect, so it is possible that the true result is 1 or even slightly more than 1, which means that there is no significant benefit.

The combined result gives a relative risk (or risk ratio) of 0.90, represented by the diamond. This represents the relative decrease in instrumental vaginal birth for those women who had a midwife-led model of care. You will recall that if the two treatments were equally effective, this ratio should be 1. Instead, it is 0.90. This means there is a 10% relative decrease in instrumental vaginal births in the midwife-led care group compared with the other models of care group. For this relative decrease of 10%, the 95% confidence intervals were 0.83 to 0.97. This is quite a narrow range, within which the true reduction is estimated to lie 95% of the time. This indicates that the true treatment effect for instrumental vaginal birth could be reduced by as much as 17% or as little as 3%. Because the 95% confidence interval does not cross 1, the line of no effect, we can be more confident with the result. If the results had been expressed as an odds ratio, they would have been very similar to the results expressed as a risk ratio (OR 0.88, 95% CI 0.80–0.96). You will recall from the previous discussion that relative risks and odds ratios are similar if the outcome is rare.

In a meta-analysis, each study does not make an equal contribution to the pooled estimate. Rather, studies are given a "weight," specified as a percentage, to reflect the amount of information that they contain. The more informative the study, the more weight it is given and the greater its contribution to the pooled estimate. The contribution to the pooled estimate of each of the studies is shown in the column labeled "Weight."

It is important when interpreting a meta-analysis to look for evidence of heterogeneity. Any differences between the individual trials in types of patients, interventions, and outcomes (clinical heterogeneity) or in the methods used in the individual trials (methodological heterogeneity) need to be considered. If the differences between trials are too great, then it may not be appropriate to pool the data in a meta-analysis. Heterogeneity can be assessed visually by examining the meta-analysis plot to see if the results of the individual trials are generally overlapping and not scattered, and also with the aid of statistical tests (Chi-squared; I-squared). A non-significant Chi-squared (Chi^2) result is indicated by a P-value greater than 0.10 and denotes that heterogeneity is not present. However, this finding needs to be interpreted together with the I-squared test. The Chi^2 test is not a robust test when the number of trials in an analysis is small and may give a non-significant result even when important heterogeneity is present. The I-squared statistic quantifies the amount of heterogeneity. If the I-squared exceeds 50%, then heterogeneity may be substantial.

A Note on Cochrane Systematic Reviews

Finding a systematic review that addresses your clinical questions is a "shortcut" in evidence-based practice. The laborious tasks of searching for, critically appraising, and synthesizing data from individual studies will already have been done by the reviewer. However, to be confident of the systematic review findings, one would need to be reassured that the review was of high quality (later in this chapter we discuss how to appraise a systematic review).

There is one major problem with systematic reviews published in paper journals. They can only be current up to the date of publication. This problem has been addressed by Cochrane. Systematic reviews published on the Cochrane Library are regularly updated as new evidence becomes available. Duplication of effort is avoided as individual review groups within Cochrane publish the titles of all systematic reviews as soon as the review process has started. The other important advantage of Cochrane Systematic Reviews is that they are required to follow the well-established, rigorous methodology of the Cochrane Collaboration, briefly outlined in Box 7.1. The primary emphasis of Cochrane has been systematic reviews looking at the effects of healthcare interventions for prevention, treatment, and rehabilitation. The scope has changed to also include systematic reviews of studies assessing diagnostic test accuracy, systematic reviews of mixed methods, overviews summarizing the evidence from several systematic reviews, and systematic reviews incorporating network meta-analyses.

SYSTEMATIC REVIEWS OF QUALITATIVE RESEARCH

Systematic reviews of qualitative research are also known as Qualitative Evidence Syntheses (QES), the preferred term of the Cochrane Qualitative and Implementation Methods Group (Booth et al., 2016). The aim of a QES is to *integrate* evidence from primary qualitative studies to develop new cumulative knowledge; an approach different from that of simply *aggregating* studies, as has been more traditional in literature reviews of qualitative research. The process of a qualitative evidence synthesis enables researchers to "go beyond" the findings of individual qualitative studies by producing something that is greater than their simple sum (Carroll et al., 2017). In doing this, outcomes may be identified that are not seen as important in a single qualitative study, and more powerful explanations can be made. It is possible for a QES to produce a nuanced, in-depth, and extremely useful picture of patient, carer, and other health systems users' experiences, beliefs, and priorities (Carroll et al., 2017).

Cochrane Reviews have predominantly concentrated on the synthesis of RCTs and cohort studies that are essential for answering questions of effectiveness. The development of approaches for QES has occurred against a backdrop of increasing demand from decision makers for evidence that goes beyond "what works," produced by such reviews. It is increasingly recognized that nursing care involves complex, multi-factorial decisions, which may require more than this original "rationalist" model of synthesis can provide (Flemming, 2007).

The terminology around QES can be confusing as it is an umbrella term. Other commonly used umbrella terms to describe the methodology include (Booth et al., 2016):

- Qualitative systematic reviews
- Qualitative evidence synthesis
- Qualitative meta-synthesis
- Qualitative research synthesis

There are over 20 different methods for qualitative synthesis (Booth et al., 2016). The most commonly used QES methods with the greatest number of exemplars are:

- Thematic synthesis (Thomas and Harden, 2008)
- Thomas and Harden's thematic synthesis includes initially coding the findings of the primary studies and then developing descriptive themes, which remain close to the primary studies. Where the quality and depth of data in the primary studies allows, this interpretation can be taken further to develop analytical themes that extend beyond the primary studies and generate a new interpretive account of the phenomenon of interest. Thematic synthesis has been used to help understand spouses' experiences of living with a partner with dementia (Egilstrod et al., 2018).
- Framework synthesis (Oliver et al., 2008) and "Best fit" framework synthesis (Carroll et al., 2011)
- The main function of a framework synthesis is to describe and interpret what is happening within a particular setting. Frameworks, or "best-fit" frameworks can be derived from the findings of a pre-existing systematic review or guideline, from a policy framework, from a pre-existing theory, or from a conceptual model. The framework guides and informs the synthesis of the qualitative research, and the approach has been used to examine the perspectives of people with venous leg ulceration symptoms and the impact of these on their health-related quality of life (Phillips et al., 2018).
- Meta-ethnography (Noblit and Hare, 1988)
- Meta-ethnography is an explicitly interpretative approach to synthesis and aims to create new understandings and theories from a body of work. Meta-ethnography has been used to explore complex questions such as why women continue to smoke in pregnancy (Flemming et al., 2015).

The choice of method to undertake a QES is predominantly driven by the review question.

Steps in a Qualitative Evidence Synthesis

The steps in a QES are very similar to those outlined earlier in this chapter for systematic reviews of quantitative studies. Within each step however, there are notable differences in approach.

DEVELOPMENT OF A PROTOCOL

The development of a protocol for the review follows a similar process to that already outlined in this chapter, with the consideration of appropriate planning of methods for a QES. Similarly, QES protocols should be registered with PROSPERO.

FORMULATING THE REVIEW QUESTION

The review question for a QES carries several important considerations, including guiding the methodology of the synthesis. Firstly, it helps to identify the focus for the review. This may be much more flexible than the very clearly defined process of formulating a fixed review question for a systematic review of quantitative research. The general "scope" of the review will need to be determined before questions are formulated (Harris et al., 2018). "Scope" refers to the kind of boundaries that will exist around the review, framing the topic of interest and mapping the existing information available (Harris et al., 2018). One of the key differences to question formulation for a quantitative review is that in a QES, although the questions may be fixed from the start of the review, they may emerge as a result of the findings from the initial review process (Booth et al., 2016).

There are various question formulation tools that can be used to help develop the question for a QES. Due to the type of questions that a QES can answer, most of the tools include some consideration of the context (i.e., setting, context, or environment) of the question being asked (Harris et al., 2018). One of the most commonly used frameworks is that of Setting, Perspective, Interest (Phenomenon of), Comparison, Evaluation (SPICE) (Booth et al., 2006). Simple question frameworks can be helpful in identifying concepts important to the review that will help construct the search strategy (Harris et al., 2018).

For the example of the QES that explored why women continue to smoke in pregnancy outlined earlier (Flemming et al., 2015), the worked example of SPICE is presented in Table 7.4.

SEARCHING FOR LITERATURE AND WHAT TO INCLUDE

The strategies for searching for literature reflect much of that outlined earlier in this chapter. Relevant electronic databases should be searched using structured search strategies, ideally developed

TABLE 7.4 ■ Worked Example of SPICE

Setting	Perspective	Interest, Phenomenon of	Comparison	Evaluation
In the community	Women who commence pregnancy as smokers	Smoking in pregnancy	None in this instance, but a comparison with women who quit smoking at the start of pregnancy could have been made	Knowledge beliefs and behaviors in relation to smoking in pregnancy

in consultation with an information specialist, to include searching of gray literature, citation searching and reference chasing (Harris et al., 2018). It is not yet clear how publication bias may operate in qualitative research, but it is possible that unpublished reports may offer a

"more extensive but less-filtered, representation of the phenomenon of interest"

HARRIS ET AL., 2018, P. 5.

Qualitative searches are, however, often iterative and require close consultation with the review team to ensure relevant studies are identified by the strategies adopted. Predominantly QES authors have used exhaustive searching (i.e., search for all available studies relevant to the focus of the review), but it is also feasible in a QES to stop searching for papers when it is deemed "saturation" has been reached, that is, when all available concepts in relation to a particular phenomenon are deemed to have been identified (Tong et al., 2012).

As with quantitative reviews, a QES generally has inclusion and exclusion criteria to guide reviewers as to what studies to include in their review and follows similar processes of identification and checking of studies suitable for inclusion between two reviewers.

ASSESSING THE METHODOLOGICAL STRENGTHS AND LIMITATIONS OF INCLUDED STUDIES

Opinion remains divided as to whether quality appraisal of studies included in a QES has value or not (Garside, 2014). Generally, however, reviewers make an assessment of study quality by identifying methodological strengths and limitations of a qualitative study (i.e., its rigor) (Noyes et al., 2018). Although rigor is different from "risk of bias assessment" undertaken in a quantitative review and is determined using different criteria, the information obtained in both cases is used to make judgments about the methodological limitations of studies included in a synthesis (Noyes et al., 2018).

The most commonly used tool in QES to assess study quality/methodological limitations is that developed by the Critical Appraisal Skills Program (CASP) (Noyes et al., 2018). The CASP qualitative research checklist criteria are presented in Chapter 4, Table 4.2.

DATA EXTRACTION AND SYNTHESIS

The approach taken to data extraction depends on the method of synthesis chosen for the review, and is quite different from that for a quantitative review. It is important to detail the study, its context, participants, methods, and approaches, and these data usually feature in the "table of included studies" of a review. Knowing the details of the participants and their context is key to the interpretation of the review's findings by users of the review.

Qualitative findings take several forms within a paper and may be in the form of quotes from participants interviewed within a primary study, sub-themes and themes presented by authors, or authors' interpretations, explanations, or theories (Noyes et al., 2018). Mostly these are found in the section labeled "Results" or "Findings," but may also be found within the discussion section of a paper.

Some of the approaches for QES are designed to extract data from the primary studies to develop descriptive-level review findings (e.g., thematic synthesis), whereas others look to develop new theory (e.g., meta-ethnography) (Noyes et al., 2018). Whichever the aim of the review, data extraction, analysis, and synthesis in a QES are iterative processes that require discussion and consultation within the review team. This is very different from the linear, sequential approach undertaken in a quantitative review (Noyes et al., 2018). Data may be extracted and coded inductively from the included studies or deductively using a predetermined framework or theory. Textual data management software can be used to help support the inductive coding of findings across the studies and the development of themes.

It is beyond the scope of this chapter to detail all the approaches to data extraction and synthesis, but the INTEGRATE-Health Technology Assessment guidance (Booth et al., 2016) and Noyes et al. paper (Noyes et al., 2018) both detail how to choose and conduct the methodology and methods for QES in an accessible way.

How Do We Report Qualitative Evidence Syntheses?

Reporting guidelines help to set standards for reporting of all types of reviews, and QES is no exception. There is one generic reporting tool for QES that has been developed: the Entrancing Transparency in Reporting the Synthesis of Qualitative Research (ENTREQ) statement. This 21-item statement guides reviewers to report the stages most commonly associated with the synthesis of qualitative health research, namely: searching and selecting qualitative research, quality appraisal, and methods for synthesizing qualitative findings (Tong et al., 2012).

Further developmental work has been undertaken to develop methodological-specific reporting guidance. The eMERGe project (http://emergeproject.org/) has developed reporting guidelines for meta-ethnography with the aim of improving the reporting of meta-ethnographies (France et al., 2015).

How Can Systematic Reviews Inform Practice?

Let us suppose that you are a nurse/midwife working in a busy prenatal clinic in an inner-city hospital. There are high rates of unemployment and social deprivation within your practice population. At the booking appointment of a young primiparous woman, she discloses that she smokes a pack of cigarettes a day. She is aware of the risks to her baby, and although she would like to stop, she is worried that she will not be able to cope if she stopped completely. She is interested in trying nicotine replacement therapy (NRT). While discussing methods of smoking cessation, you realize that you are no longer confident with up-to-date evidence around smoking cessation and NRT. You give her some leaflets on stopping smoking, and the woman agrees to be referred to the smoking cessation counselor for specialist support.

This realization has prompted you to search for the evidence around available treatments for smoking cessation in pregnancy. You start by searching on the Cochrane Library. A search on "smoking cessation" AND pregnancy, restricted to the title, abstract, and key words, yields seven systematic reviews in the Cochrane Database of Systematic Reviews. One of the abstracts, entitled "Pharmacological interventions for promoting smoking cessation during pregnancy" (Coleman et al., 2015), seems relevant to your question. The "criteria for considering studies" shows the types of studies eligible for inclusion in the review: RCTs of pregnant women who smoked, in which the interventions included pharmacotherapies (including NRT, varenicline, and bupropion), other medications, ENDS (electronic nicotine delivery systems), or e-cigarettes when used for smoking cessation in pregnancy. The main outcome assessed was smoking cessation in pregnancy. The review group divided the interventions into placebo-controlled trials and non–placebo-controlled trials.

The review included nine trials that enrolled 2210 pregnant smokers: eight trials of NRT and one trial of bupropion as adjuncts to behavioral support/CBT. The results are illustrated in Table 7.5. The pooled relative risk for this group was 1.41 (95% CI 1.03–1.93). As you can see, the combined result indicated by the diamond does not cross the vertical line of "no effect," which means the combined result is significant. However, the pooled relative risk for the subgroup of placebo-controlled trials provided a lower RR of 1.28 (95% CI 0.99–1.66), with the confidence interval just crossing the line of no effect and therefore not significant. For the subgroup of non-placebo

TABLE 7.5 ■ Pharmacological Interventions for Smoking Cessation in Pregnancy*

Study or Subgroup	NRT Events	NRT Total	Control Events	Control Total	Weight	Risk Ratio M-H, Random, 95% CI	Risk Ratio M-H, Random, 95% CI
1.1.1 Placebo-controlled trials							
Oncken 2008	18	100	14	94	18.1%	1.21 [0.64, 2.29]	
Coleman 2012	49	521	40	529	33.5%	1.24 [0.83, 1.86]	
Berlin 2014	25	203	19	199	21.8%	1.29 [0.73, 2.27]	
Wisborg 2000	22	124	17	126	20.8%	1.31 [0.73, 2.35]	
Kapur 2001	4	17	0	13	1.2%	7.00 [0.41, 119.46]	
Subtotal (95% CI)		965		961	95.3%	1.28 [0.99, 1.66]	
Total events	118		90				
Heterogeneity: Tau^2 = 0.00; Chi^2 = 1.45, df = 4 (P = 0.84); I^2 = 0%							
Test for overall effect: Z = 1.87 (P = 0.06)							
1.1.2 Non Placebo-controlled trials							
Hotham 2006	3	20	0	20	1.1%	7.00 [0.38, 127.32]	
Pollak 2007	17	122	1	59	2.4%	8.22 [1.12, 60.31]	
El-Mohandes 2013	5	26	0	26	1.2%	11.00 [0.64, 189.31]	
Subtotal (95% CI)		168		105	4.7%	8.51 [2.05, 35.28]	
Total events	25		1				
Heterogeneity: Tau^2 = 0.00; Chi^2 = 0.05, df = 2 (P = 0.98); I^2 = 0%							
Test for overall effect: Z = 2.95 (P = 0.003)							
Total (95% CI)		1133		1066	100.0%	1.41 [1.03, 1.93]	
Total events	143		91				
Heterogeneity: Tau^2 = 0.03; Chi^2 = 8.51, df = 7 (P = 0.29); I^2 = 18%							
Test for overall effect: Z = 2.15 (P = 0.03)							
Test for subgroup differences: Chi^2 = 6.59, df = 1 (P = 0.01); I^2 = 84.8%							

0.1 0.2 0.5 1 2 5 10
Favors control   Favors NRT

*The outcome is smoking cessation in pregnancy.
Copyright Cochrane Library, with Permission.

RCTs, there was a stronger positive effect of NRT (RR 8.51, 95% CI 2.05–35.28). The evidence suggests that when potentially biased, non-placebo RCTs are excluded from analyses, NRT is not as effective. Finally, you want to look for evidence of heterogeneity. On examination of the forest plot in Table 7.5, it is clear that the majority of the trials fall to the right side with confidence intervals overlapping. The P-value of 0.29 for the Chi^2 test indicates that no heterogeneity is present. Finally, you are reassured by a value of 18% for the I-squared statistic, again indicating minimal heterogeneity. You conclude that it was appropriate for the eight trials to have been pooled in a meta-analysis.

The quality of the review is appraised using the checklist in Box 7.2, adapted from the Critical Appraisal Skills Programme (CASP) 2010 systematic review checklist. This checklist helps the reviewer to distinguish between literature and systematic reviews, and to assess the rigor of the methodology used. The latter point is particularly important as there is evidence of considerable variation in quality of systematic reviews. The term "systematic review" may have been applied to something inferior.

The objectives of this review clearly lay out the research question, and the right type of study was included. A detailed search strategy has been prepared within the collaborative review group responsible for the review, and this is comprehensive. Specific inclusion and exclusion criteria are reported, and the quality of the included studies is clearly described. The meta-analysis addressed appropriate comparisons and was easy to understand. The conclusions of the review appear appropriate and supported by the evidence obtained in the review:

> "NRT used in pregnancy for smoking cessation increases smoking cessation rates measured in late pregnancy by approximately 40%. There is evidence, suggesting that when potentially-biased, non-placebo RCTs are excluded from analyses, NRT is no more effective than placebo."

Finally, you look at the population characteristics of the women in the RCTs: they are all pregnant women who were at least 16 years of age; smoking between 1 and 15 cigarettes a day; and

---

BOX 7.2 ■ Checklist for Appraising Systematic Reviews

1. Did the review address a clearly focused question?
2. Did the authors look for the right type of papers?
3. Do you think all the important, relevant studies were included?
4. Did the review's authors do enough to assess the quality of the included studies?
5. If the results of the reviews have been combined, was it reasonable to do so?
6. What are the overall results of the review?
7. How precise are these results?
8. Can the results be applied to the local population?
9. Were all important outcomes considered?
10. Are the benefits worth the harms and costs?

©CASP Checklist: 10 Questions to Help You Make Sense of a Systematic Review.

---

were recruited into trials in Australia, Canada, Denmark, the UK, and the US. These populations appear similar to the population of women seen in your prenatal clinic. You feel reassured that the results will be applicable in your setting.

You now have the evidence for the effectiveness of NRT use in pregnancy, however, you are uncertain as to how acceptable NRT use is to women who are pregnant and are looking to quit smoking. You search in CINAHL using the terms "smoking in pregnancy," "systematic review," and "qualitative" to try and find a qualitative evidence synthesis of smoking in pregnancy and identify a review that explores the barriers and facilitators to smoking cessation experienced by women in pregnancy and after childbirth (Flemming et al., 2015). Within the review, you identify that only one study included in the review has looked at the women's view of NRT.

The CASP systematic review checklist (see Box 7.2) was not developed with QES in mind, and a number of the questions are not that appropriate to the methods used within a QES. Currently, there is no critical appraisal tool that has been developed to appraise the quality of QES. One alternative is to use the ENTREQ reporting guidance for QES, discussed earlier, to determine whether the authors have included all they should have in their report of the review. This does not determine quality of process, but can demonstrate that necessary processes were reported. On reading the review again, you discover that the authors reported the review in accordance with the ENTREQ guidance, and so you feel reassured that the detail you require from the review is present within it.

The findings from the two reviews you have identified leads you to conclude that you know that NRT is an effective intervention to assist women to quit smoking, but there is no clear evidence about how acceptable its use is with pregnant women.

You decide therefore to introduce the idea of NRT when approaching the subject of quitting smoking in pregnancy with women, but know that you will need to determine how the risks and benefits of NRT are perceived by women on a case-by-case basis.

Summary

It will be clear by now that systematic reviews are an important element of evidence-based practice. When assessing the effectiveness of an intervention, a systematic review of RCTs is considered "gold standard" evidence. When seeking explanation of people's experiences, views, and values of health care, illness, services, and so on, then a systematic review of qualitative research is the most appropriate form of review to read. As a research activity, systematic reviews are important and need to be performed thoroughly. This chapter has described the basic methodology of two main types of reviews. All practitioners will need to use systematic reviews, so it is important to understand the methods, how the results are presented, and to be able to judge the quality of reviews to assess whether their results are valid.

Exercise

We encourage you to consolidate your learning by undertaking the exercise available at http://evolve.elsevier.com/Craig/evidence/

Acknowledgement

We thank Rosalind Smyth, whose contributions to previous editions have helped to inform this chapter.

References

Booth, A., 2006. Clear and present questions: formulating questions for evidence based practice. 24. Library Hi Tech., pp. 355–368.

Booth, A., 2016. Searching for qualitative research for inclusion in systematic reviews: a structured methodological review. Syst. Rev. 5 (1), 74.

Booth, A., Noyes, J., Flemming, K., et al., 2016. Guidance on choosing qualitative evidence synthesis methods for use in health technology assessments of complex interventions. Available from: http://www.integrate-hta.eu/downloads/ (Accessed 20.04.18.).

Carroll, C., 2017. Qualitative evidence synthesis to improve implementation of clinical guidelines. BMJ 356, j80. https://doi.org/10.1136/bmj.j80.

Carroll, C., Booth, A., Cooper, K., 2011. A worked example of "best fit" framework synthesis: a systematic review of views concerning the taking of some potential chemo-preventive agents. BMC Med. Res. Methodol. 11 (1), 29.

Coleman, T., Chamberlain, C., Davey, M.A., Cooper, S.E., Leonardi-Bee, J., 2015. Pharmacological interventions for promoting smoking cessation during pregnancy. Cochrane Database Syst. Rev. 12 (9), CD010078. https://doi.org/10.1002/14651858.CD010078.pub2.

Critical Appraisal Skills Programme, 2018. CASP (Systematic Review) Checklist. Available from: https://casp-uk.net/casp-tools-checklists/ (Accessed 12.11.18.).

Critical Appraisal Skills Programme, 2018. CASP (Qualitative) Checklist. Available from: https://casp-uk.net/casp-tools-checklists/ (Accessed 12.11.18.).

Crowley, P., 1996. Prophylactic corticosteroids for preterm birth (Cochrane Review). Cochrane Database Syst. Rev. 1, CD000065. https://doi.org/10.1002/14651858.CD000065*.

Deeks, J.J., Higgins, J.P.T., Altman, D.G., 2011. Chapter 9: analysing data and undertaking meta-analyses. In: Higgins, J.P.T., Green, S. (Eds.), Cochrane Handbook for Systematic Reviews of Interventions Version 5.1.0 (updated March 2011). The Cochrane Collaboration. Available from: www.handbook.cochrane.org (Accessed 12.04.18.).

Downe, S., Finlayson, K., Melvin, C., Spiby, H., Ali, S., Diggle, P., et al., 2015. Self-hypnosis for intrapartum pain management in pregnant nulliparous women: a randomised controlled trial of clinical effectiveness. BJOG 122 (9), 1226–1234. https://doi.org/10.1111/1471-0528.13433.

Dwan, K., Gamble, C., Williamson, P.R., Kirkham, J., the Reporting Bias Group, 2013. Systematic review of the empirical evidence of study publication bias and outcome reporting bias—an updated review. PLoS One 8 (7), e66844. https://doi.org/10.1371/journal.pone.0066844 PMCID: PMC3702538.

Egilstrod, B., Ravn, M.B., Petersen, K.S., 2018. Living with a partner with dementia: a systematic review and thematic synthesis of spouses' lived experiences of changes in their everyday lives. Aging Ment. Health 6 (1), 1–10.

Flemming, K., 2007. The synthesis of qualitative research and evidence based nursing. Evid. Based Nurs. 10, 68–71.

Flemming, K., McCaughan, D., Angus, K., Graham, H., 2015. Qualitative systematic review: barriers and facilitators to smoking cessation experienced by women in pregnancy and following childbirth. J. Adv. Nurs. 71 (6), 1210–1226. https://doi.org/10.1111/jan.12580.

France, E.F., Ring, N., Noyes, J., Maxwell, M., Jepson, R., Duncan, E., et al., 2015. Protocol-developing meta-ethnography reporting guidelines (eMERGe). BMC Med. Res. Methodol. 15, 103.

Francis, D.K., Smith, J., Saljuqi, T., Watling, R.M., 2015. Oral protein calorie supplementation for children with chronic disease. Cochrane Database Syst. Rev. 5, CD001914. https://doi.org/10.1002/14651858.CD001914.pub2.

Garside, R., 2014. Should we appraise the quality of qualitative research reports for systematic reviews, and if so, how? Innovat. Eur. J. Soc. Sci. Res. 27, 67e79.

Green, S., Higgins, J.P.T., 2011. Chapter 2: Preparing a Cochrane review. In: Higgins, J.P.T., Green, S. (Eds.), Cochrane Handbook for Systematic Reviews of Interventions Version 5.1.0 (updated March 2011). The Cochrane Collaboration. Available from: www.handbook.cochrane.org (Accessed 14.04.18.).

Harris, J.L., Booth, A., Cargo, M., Hannes, K., Harden, A., Flemming, K., et al., 2018. Cochrane Qualitative and Implementation Methods Group guidance series—paper 6: methods for question formulation, searching and protocol development for qualitative evidence synthesis. J. Clin. Epidemiol. 97, 39–48. https://doi.org/10.1016/j.jclinepi.2017.10.023.

Higgins, J.P.T., Altman, D.G., Sterne, J.A.C., 2011. Assessing risk of bias in included studies. In: Higgins, J.P.T., Green, S. (Eds.), Cochrane Handbook for Systematic Reviews of Interventions Version 5.1.0 (updated March 2011). The Cochrane Collaboration. Chapter 8: Available from: www.cochrane-handbook.org (Accessed 15.04.18.).

Knipschild, P., 1995. Some examples of systematic reviews. In: Chalmers, I., Altman, D.G. (Eds.), Systematic Reviews. BMJ Publishing, London, pp. 9–16.

Ma, Y., Dong, M., Zhou, K., Mita, C., Liu, J., Wayne, P.M., 2016. Publication trends in acupuncture research: a 20-year bibliometric analysis based on PubMed. PLoS One 11 (12), e0168123. https://doi.org/10.1371/journal.pone.0168123. eCollection 2016.

McFadden, A., Gavine, A., Renfrew, M.J., Wade, A., Buchanan, P., Taylor, J.L., et al., 2017. Support for healthy breastfeeding mothers with healthy term babies. Cochrane Database Syst. Rev. 2, CD001141. https://doi.org/10.1002/14651858.CD001141.pub5.

Noblit, G.W., Hare, R.D., 1988. Meta-Ethnography: Synthesizing Qualitative Studies. Sage Publications, Newbury Park.

Noyes, J., Booth, A., Flemming, K., Garside, R., Harden, A., Lewin, S., et al., 2018. Cochrane Qualitative and Implementation Methods Group guidance paper 3: methods for assessing methodological limitations, data extraction and synthesis, and confidence in synthesized qualitative findings. J. Clin. Epidemiol. 97, 49–58. https://doi.org/10.1016/ j.jclinepi.2017.06.020.

Oliver, S., Rees, R., Clarke-Jones, L., et al., 2008. A multidimensional conceptual framework for analysing public involvement in health services research. Health Expect. 11 (4), 72–84. https://doi.org/10.1111/j.1369-7625.2007.00476.x.

Pauling, L., 1986. How to Live Long and Feel Better. Freeman, New York.

Phillips, P., Lumley, E., Duncan, R., Aber, A., Woods, H.B., Jones, G.L., Michaels, J.A., 2018. A systematic review of qualitative research into people's experiences of living with venous leg ulcers. J. Adv. Nurs. 74 (3), 550–563.

PROSPERO, International prospective register of systematic reviews. Available from: https://www.crd.york.ac.uk/prospero/ (Accessed 17.3.18.).

Sandall, J., Soltani, H., Gates, S., Shennan, A., Devane, D., 2016. Midwife-led continuity models versus other models of care for childbearing women. Cochrane Database Syst. Rev. 4, CD004667. https://doi.org/10.1002/14651858.CD004667.pub5.*

Schünemann, H., Brożek, J., Guyatt, G., Oxman, A. (Eds.), 2013. GRADE handbook for grading quality of evidence and strength of recommendations. Updated October 2013. The GRADE Working Group. Available from: guidelinedevelopment.org/handbook (Accessed 02.04.18.).

Thomas, J., Harden, A., 2008. Methods for the thematic synthesis of qualitative research in systematic reviews. BMC Med. Res. Methodol. 8, 45.

Tong, A., Flemming, K., McInnes, E., Oliver, S., Craig, J., 2012. Enhancing transparency in reporting the synthesis of qualitative research: ENTREQ. BMC Med. Res. Methodol. 12 (1), 181 PMID: 23185978.

---

* Cochrane Reviews are regularly updated as new information becomes available and in response to comments and criticism. The reader should consult The Cochrane Library for the latest version of a Cochrane Review. Information on The Cochrane Library can be found at https://www.cochranelibrary.com/

Further Reading

Cochrane. Available from: http://www.cochrane.org/ (Accessed 20.04.18.).

Cochrane Qualitative and Implementation Methods Group. Available from: http://methods.cochrane.org/qi/ (Accessed 20.04.18.).

GRADEpro, G.D.T., 2015. GRADEpro Guideline Development Tool [Software]. McMaster University (developed by Evidence Prime, Inc.). Available from: https://gradepro.org/.

Hannes, K., Lockwood, C., 2011. Synthesizing Qualitative Research: Choosing the Right Approach. John Wiley & Sons, Chicester, West Sussex.

The Cochrane Collaboration. In: Higgins, J.P.T., Green, S. (Eds.), 2011. Cochrane Handbook for Systematic Reviews of Interventions Version 5.1.0 (updated March 2011) Available from: www.handbook.cochrane.org (Accessed 20.04.18.).

Saini, M., Shlonsky, A., 2012. Systematic Synthesis of Qualitative Research (Pocket Guides to Social Work Research Methods). Oxford University Press, Oxford.

Schünemann, H., Brożek, J., Guyatt, G., Oxman, A. (Eds.), 2013. GRADE handbook for grading quality of evidence and strength of recommendations. Updated October 2013. The GRADE Working Group. Available from: guidelinedevelopment.org/handbook (Accessed 15.04.18.).

Centre for Reviews and Dissemination, 2009. Systematic Reviews: CRD's Guidance for Undertaking Reviews in Health Care. University of York NHS Centre for Reviews & Dissemination: Heslington, York.

CHAPTER 8

Evidence-Based Guidelines

Dawn Dowding ■ Arlene Smaldone

Introduction

Clinical practice guidelines are one of the main ways in which knowledge generated through research can be implemented into clinical practice. Clinical practice guidelines provide a full range of management options for a particular problem or condition, normally including an assessment of the benefits and harms of alternative care options. They are ideally informed by high-quality systematic reviews (which may include meta-analyses), but also include evidence from other sources when such reviews are not available. Through their explicit rating of the quality or robustness of the evidence on which recommendations are based, they can assist health professionals and patients in healthcare decision-making and delivery of care.

Over the past 30 years, development of clinical practice guidelines has proliferated, often with multiple guidelines addressing the same clinical condition. Although the Institute of Medicine report, *Clinical Practice Guidelines We Can Trust* (Institute of Medicine, 2011), recommends that guideline developers adhere to eight essential standards to assure guideline trustworthiness, there is wide variation in the overall quality of clinical guidelines that are produced within and between different countries (Duda et al., 2017; Holmer et al., 2013).

As the largest component of the healthcare workforce, active participation by nurses in both the development and implementation of guidelines is critical. However, nurses often report that they have problems adhering to guideline recommendations for care. An integrative review (Jun et al., 2016) of 16 studies conducted in 7 countries found that nurses reported adhering to guidelines between 53% (Forberg et al., 2014) and 83.4% (Ebben et al., 2015) of the time.

Individual-level barriers to guideline use included attitudes such as lack of motivation and perceptions that guidelines reduced clinician autonomy and critical thinking, impaired a nurse's ability to provide individualized care, and provided little to no benefit, particularly if guidelines were not used by physicians at their setting. In contrast, when nurses perceived that guidelines were useful (e.g., assisted nurses who were less experienced, reduced medication errors, or improved processes of care and patient outcomes), they were more likely not only to use guidelines but also encourage their use by other nurses. Although the majority of nurses who participated in the included studies reported moderate to high general knowledge regarding guidelines, they often reported guideline formats as cumbersome and not readily available when they needed to refer to them. Nurses also reported that many guidelines were available for the same clinical situation, and it was difficult to distinguish which guideline to use. On a systems level, the most frequently reported barriers included time, staffing, and logistical issues. However, when guidelines were endorsed by peers, integrated within the electronic medical system, and/or available via either the Internet or an institution's intranet, guideline use was facilitated.

Clearly, research to date suggests that integration of clinical practice guidelines into nursing practice is not optimal, and there is room for improvement. Given this context, the purpose of this chapter is to provide you with the resources to know how to locate clinical guidelines, appraise the guidelines for quality, determine the level of evidence that informs a given practice recommendation, and identify best practices for guideline implementation within your clinical practice setting.

How to Access Clinical Guidelines

The way in which guidelines are developed varies across countries (Bhaumik, 2017). In some countries, guidelines are developed by individual professional organizations and/or agencies with a centralized agency designated to coordinate guidelines. In the US, the National Guideline Clearinghouse (https://www.guideline.gov), a database updated weekly by the Agency for Healthcare Research and Quality, serves as a repository for guidelines developed by many professional organizations (National Guideline Clearinghouse, 2012). Because the process of guideline development among professional organizations lacks a unified approach, the methodology, guideline group composition, and potential conflicts of interest of guideline developers may vary widely. Since 1998, the National Guideline Clearinghouse, funded federally through the Agency for Healthcare Research and Quality (AHRQ), has summarized key recommendations of each guideline and the methods by which they were developed, thus enabling the user to make side-by-side comparisons of guidelines addressing the same topic. Due to federal budget cuts to the AHRQ, the National Guidelines Clearinghouse ceased operations on July 16, 2018. Although planning has not been finalized at this time, the ECRI Institute, a nonprofit agency that provided oversight to the work of the National Guidelines Clearinghouse since its inception, plans to replace the website with a subscription-based website and run it privately (see www.ecri.org/guidelines for more information).

In other countries, a central agency is responsible for guideline development. For example, in England and Scotland there are the National Institute for Health and Care Excellence (NICE) ("Improving health and social care through evidence-based guidance") (NICE, 2018) and the Scottish Intercollegiate Guidelines Network (SIGN) (Shaku and Tsutsumi, 2016). Methodology for guideline development is standardized by NICE and SIGN, and full access to their guidelines is available via their respective websites. Table 8.1 provides detail regarding structure of guideline development and access across 11 high-income countries in North America, Europe, and Oceania ranked by the Commonwealth Fund by level of health system performance (Schneider et al., 2017).

To try and ensure that guidelines are of good quality, a number of organizations have published standards for guideline developers (Qaseem et al., 2012; NICE, 2014; Dahlqvist Jonsson et al.,

TABLE 8.1 ■ Clinical Practice Guideline Development Among Select High-Income Countries by 2017 Commonwealth Fund Overall Health System Ranking

Rank	Country	Guideline Development Responsibility	Central or Coordinating Agency	Website and Guideline Accessibility
1	United Kingdom	Central agency	NICE – England and Wales SIGN – Scotland	https://www.nice.org.uk/guidance • full public access • organized by disease/condition, population group, etc. http://www.sign.ac.uk/our-guidelines.html • organized by publication date
2	Australia	Multiple organizations with central coordination	NHRMC*	https://www.clinicalguidelines.gov.au/ • full public access with additional provider and patient resources
3	Netherlands	Multiple organizations with central coordination	Council for Quality of Care	Royal Dutch Society for Physical Therapy (KNGF) guidelines • all available in English
4	New Zealand	Central agency	New Zealand Guidelines Group	https://www.health.govt.nz/search/results/guidelines?f%5B0%5D=im_field_publication_type%3A26#find-by-region
4	Norway	Central agency	Norwegian Directorate of the Health Services*	http://www.helsebiblioteket.no/om-oss/english?emneside=true • free access to more than 400 Norwegian clinical guidelines, scoring tools and patient information leaflets
6	Sweden	Central agency	Swedish National Board of Health and Welfare	http://www.socialstyrelsen.se/nationalguidelines • full access to guideline summaries • all available in English
6	Switzerland	Multiple organizations with no central coordination	No national guideline agency	No website
8	Germany	Multiple organizations with central coordination	Association of Scientific Medical Societies in Germany	http://www.awmf.org/en/awmf-online-portal-for-scientific-medicine/awmf-news.html

9	Canada	Multiple organizations with central coordination	Canadian Medical Association*	Clinical Practice Guideline Infobase: https://www.cma.ca/En/Pages/clinical-practice-guidelines.aspx • includes guidelines developed in Canada, England, and the US • full public access to guidelines produced in Canada with additional provider and patient resources • all available in English; some available in French
10	France	Multiple organizations with central coordination	Haute Authorité de Sauté	https://www.has-sante.fr/portail/jcms/r_1455081/en/home-page?portal=r_1455081 • public access to guidelines • includes guideline development group by discipline and guideline methodology • available in French and English
11	United States	Multiple organizations with central coordination	National Guideline Clearinghouse*	• guideline summaries organized by clinical specialty enabling comparison of up to 3 guideline summaries • systematic comparisons of guidelines that address similar topics highlighting areas of agreement and differences between recommendations • access to full guideline varies by developer • National Guideline Clearinghouse ceased operations on July 16, 2018, due to lack of federal funding. As of September 2018, access to guideline summaries is not available (further information at: https://www.ecri.org/Pages/ECRI_guidelines.aspx)

NICE, National Institute for Health and Care Excellence; *SIGN*, Scottish Intercollegiate Guidelines Network; *NHRMC*, National Health and Medical Research Council.
Responsibility for both developing guidelines and approving guidelines developed by others.

2015; Ransohoff and Sox, 2013). To be considered high quality, a guideline must meet eight standards (Institute of Medicine, 2011) including the following:

- Transparent guideline development and funding
- Minimal potential conflict of interest of guideline developers
- Broad composition of guideline developers by discipline and expertise including representation by those affected by the condition
- High-quality systematic reviews as the guideline foundation
- Level of evidence and degree of certainty provided for each guideline recommendation
- Action recommended by the guideline fully described as well as the indications for use
- Process of external review by a full spectrum of stakeholders including the public before guideline implementation
- Timeline for guideline updating

One of the main problems with clinical guidelines is that the process for updating guideline recommendations is unclear. In general, these processes are poorly described in the methodologies used by guideline developers (Vernooij et al., 2014) and a strong evidence base regarding best practices for monitoring both the need for and the actual updating of clinical practice guidelines is lacking (Martinez Garcia et al., 2012). This means that as a guideline user you need to first assess a guideline to make sure it is up to date. A general rule of thumb is that a guideline should be routinely re-evaluated to make sure that it is up to date at least every 3 years (Shekelle et al., 2012). Guidelines older than 5 years should be used with caution because as many as one-half may be out of date (Shekelle et al., 2001). For example, Neuman et al. reviewed the type and extent of changes made to recommendations of 11 American College of Cardiology/American Heart Association guidelines after their update by guideline developers (Neuman et al., 2014). Across the cardiology guidelines examined, the majority of recommendations were retained after updating. However, 2.9% to 12.7% of recommendations were either downgraded or reversed, and 2.2% to 69.2% of recommendations were omitted from the updated guideline, illustrating the critical importance of guideline updating to reflect current research.

The amount of time that any one specific guideline recommendation will remain current varies both within and across guidelines. A guideline requires updating when there is new evidence regarding current therapeutic options, benefits, and harms of existing therapies, or changes in either outcomes deemed important, values placed on outcomes, or resources available for health care (Clark et al., 2006; Uhlig et al., 2016). Specific recommendations regarding best practices for guideline updating may be found in "Developing NICE Guidelines: The manual" (NICE, 2014).

Appraising Guideline Quality

Before you can implement a guideline into clinical practice, you need to appraise it for quality. Often there may be more than one guideline for a particular condition or aspect of care available, and the methods for their development vary across professional organizations. There are a number of appraisal tools available for guideline appraisal. A systematic review of 40 instruments published between 1995 and 2009 identified the Appraisal of Guidelines for Research and Evaluation II (AGREE II) as the most comprehensively validated instrument (Siering et al., 2013). AGREE II has been used to compare the quality of clinical guidelines in a number of areas of practice important to nursing, such as nutritional support for critically ill adults (Fuentes Padilla et al., 2016), pharmaceutical management to maintain glycemic control (Holmer et al., 2013), glycemic targets for adults with type 2 diabetes (Qaseem et al., 2018), and prevention of *Clostridium difficile* infection (Lytvyn et al., 2016). For each area of practice, between 5 (Lytvyn et al., 2016) and 24 (Holmer et al., 2013) guidelines met inclusion criteria; AGREE II domain scores were lowest for editorial independence, applicability, and stakeholder involvement in guideline development.

AGREE II is a 23-item instrument that measures six quality domains for clinical guidelines: Scope and Purpose, Stakeholder Involvement, Rigor of Development, Clarity of Presentation, Applicability, and Editorial Independence. Responses for each item may range from 1 (item poorly reported or information is absent from the guideline) to 7 (exceptional) (Brouwers et al., 2010). After item completion, the user is asked to rate the guideline's overall quality (scale from 1 to 7) and whether the guideline is recommended for use. The AGREE II user manual provides detailed instructions for calculation of scores for each domain area (this is available along with online training tools on the AGREE II website at https://www.agreetrust.org). Although specific guidance is provided for rating items 1 to 23, the two overall assessment ratings (overall quality and recommendation) are more subjective. A systematic review of examining how AGREE II users complete the two overall assessments suggests that although a consistent approach to overall assessment rating is lacking, guideline appraisers frequently use the mean of AGREE II domain scores with particular attention to domains 3 (Rigor of Development) and 5 (Applicability) as the basis for decision-making (Hoffmann-Eβer et al., 2017, 2018).

In addition to the AGREE II instrument, there is also the option to sign up to the My AGREE PLUS platform. This enables you to either appraise guidelines individually or contribute to group appraisals. Importantly, domain scores of guidelines appraised using My AGREE PLUS are automatically calculated. We have used the group appraisal process via My AGREE PLUS as a learning opportunity for doctoral-level nursing students to familiarize themselves with AGREE II and establish basic guideline-appraisal competency.

Table 8.2 summarizes findings of our AGREE II appraisal of a guideline developed by the American Association of Clinical Endocrinologists (Handelsman et al., 2015). The guideline was chosen because it addresses an important clinical question, glycemic targets for individuals with type 2 diabetes, affects approximately 16 million globally, has broad practice implications, and was one of six current guidelines addressing this clinical issue (Qaseem et al., 2018). Based on our appraisal, our overall guideline rating was 3 on a scale from 1 to 7, and, at best, we would only cautiously recommend the guideline with modifications. It is worth noting that while diabetes care espouses multidisciplinary team management with active patient engagement, only endocrinologists were involved in guideline development. Further, the guideline failed to consider barriers and facilitators and estimation of resources that might affect successful implementation of the guideline in practice settings Although our AGREE II domain scores vary a bit from those of Qaseem (Qaseem et al., 2018), the domain scores with both highest and lowest ratings are similar. It is important to recognize that appraisal is limited to the methodology on which the recommendation is based, not the specific guideline recommendations.

Guideline Recommendations and Degree of Certainty

After guideline appraisal and the decision that the guideline is trustworthy, the next step is to examine its recommendations. A guideline usually contains multiple recommendations for practice. In one study of 42 SIGN guidelines (Baird and Lawrence, 2014), the number of recommendations per guideline ranged between 9 and 158. Each recommendation should provide the level of evidence on which the recommendation is based and the degree of certainty for the recommendation. More than 100 grading systems are available to guideline developers to rate the strength of recommendations (Maymone et al., 2014). Therefore it is important that guideline users be knowledgeable about the system by which evidence is categorized and degree of certainty is established, often a challenging task because appraisal systems differ by guideline developer.

In countries where a central agency is responsible for guideline development such as in England and Scotland, a consistent method is employed for all guidelines developed within that country. For example, SIGN guidelines rank evidence level on a scale ranging between 1++ (highest

TABLE 8.2 ■ Guideline Appraisal Exemplar of Diabetes Guideline Using AGREE II

Domain/Domain Score	Item	Where to Look in the Guideline	Item Rating (1–7)	
			Rater 1	Rater 2
Scope and purpose 58%	1. Overall guideline objectives specifically described.	Opening paragraphs	7	7
	2. Health questions of guideline specifically described.	Opening paragraphs	7	4
	3. Population for whom guideline intended specifically described.	Opening paragraphs	1	1
	4. Guideline development group includes participation from all relevant professional groups.	Methods, Guideline panel member list, Acknowledgements, Appendices	1	2
Stakeholder involvement 28%	5. Views and preferences of target population have been sought.	Methods, Guideline panel member list, External review, Target population perspectives	1	1
	6. Guideline target users clearly defined.	Opening paragraphs	4	7
Rigor of development 49%	7. Systematic methods to search for evidence used.	Methods, Literature search strategy, Appendices	1	2
	8. Criteria for selecting evidence clearly described.	Methods, Literature search, Inclusion/exclusion criteria, Appendices	1	1
	9. Body of evidence strengths and limitations clearly described.	Evidence quality tables, Results, Discussion	5	4
	10. Methods for formulating recommendations clearly described.	Methods, Guideline development process	7	3
	11. Health benefits, side effects, and risks considered in formulating recommendations.	Methods, Interpretation, Discussion, Recommendations	5	7
Clarity of presentation 50%	12. Explicit link between recommendations and supporting evidence.	Recommendations, Key evidence	7	7
	13. Before publication, guideline externally reviewed by experts.	Methods, Results, Interpretation, Acknowledgements	7	4

TABLE 8.2 ■ Guideline Appraisal Exemplar of Diabetes Guideline Using AGREE II—cont'd

Domain/Domain Score	Item	Where to Look in the Guideline	Item Rating (1–7)	
	14. Procedure for updating guideline provided.	Methods, Guideline update, Date of guideline	1	1
	15. Specific and unambiguous recommendations.	Recommendations, Executive summary	4	7
	16. Different options for management of condition or health issue clearly presented.	Executive summary, Recommendations, Discussion, Treatment options, Treatment alternatives	4	5
	17. Key recommendations easily identifiable.	Executive summary, Conclusions, Recommendations	1	3
Applicability 4%	18. Facilitators and barriers to guideline application described.	Barriers, Guideline utilization, Quality indicators	1	1
	19. Advice and/or tools on how guideline recommendations can be put into practice provided.	Tools, Resources, Implementation, Appendices	1	3
	20. Potential resource implications of applying guideline recommendations considered.	Methods, Cost utility, Cost effectiveness, Acquisition costs, Implications for budgets	1	1
	21. Monitoring and/or auditing criteria presented.	Recommendations, Quality indicators, Audit criteria	1	1
Editorial independence 58%	22. Funding body views have not influenced guideline content.	Disclaimer, Funding source	1	4
	23. Guideline development group member competing interests recorded and addressed.	Methods, Conflicts of interest, Guideline panel, Appendix	6	7
Overall assessment 3	Overall quality of guideline rated between 1 (lowest quality) and 7 (highest quality)		3	3
1 No 1 Yes with Modifications	Guideline recommended for use: Yes, Yes with modifications, No		No	Yes/Mod

From Handelsman, Y., Bloomgarden, Z.T., Grunberger, G., Umpierrez, G., Zimmerman, R.S., Bailey, T.S., et al., 2015. American Association of Clinical Endocrinologists and American College of Endocrinology clinical practice guidelines for developing a diabetes mellitus comprehensive care plan. Endocr. Pract. 21 (Suppl 1), 1–87. https://doi.org/10.4158/EP15672.GL

Note: Each domain score calculated as (obtained score – minimum possible score) divided by (maximum possible score – minimum possible score).

ranking, based on high-quality meta-analyses or systematic reviews of randomized controlled trials or individual studies of randomized controlled design rated as having low risk of bias) and 4 (lowest ranking, based on expert opinion) (Baird and Lawrence, 2014). Based on the evidence, recommendations are categorized between A (highest level of recommendation) and D (lowest level of recommendation). A platform, Guidelines Learning, available on the SIGN website (https://www.guidelinesfornurses.co.uk/guidelines-learning) enables individuals to stay up to date on current SIGN guidelines and accrue continuing education credit by completing modules on guideline recommendations in over 20 clinical practice areas.

In England, all NICE guidelines are developed using the same methodology. Since 2007, all NICE guideline developers have used the Grading of Recommendation Assessment, Development and Evaluation (GRADE) method (Thornton et al., 2013). Different from other systems that confine ratings to the level of evidence, GRADE incorporates the values and preferences of patients and society at large into its rating system (Dijkers, 2013). Beginning with a well-formulated PICO question, users of GRADE identify, evaluate, and summarize existing evidence, focusing on outcomes of importance; appraise the study quality to determine level of confidence in the treatment effect; and solicit patient values and preferences to determine the tradeoff between risks and benefits. From this process, guideline recommendations are developed.

Important to the GRADE method is consideration of not only the study design but also the potential risk of bias on which the evidence is generated. Using this approach, evidence from a well-designed cohort study of high quality with precise results may be upgraded. Quality of evidence supporting a recommendation may range from high quality, where additional research is unlikely to alter the level of confidence in the estimate of effect, to very low quality, where the estimated effect is very uncertain. Strength of the recommendation is based on a number of factors: the balance between risk and potential harm, evidence quality, patient values and preferences, and treatment cost. Strength may range from strongly in favor (benefits outweigh the potential harms) to weak, where the level of benefits and potential harms are similar in scope (Maymone et al., 2014). A wide variety of resources including the GRADE handbook, computer software *(GRADEpro GDT),* and workshops are available to those interested in learning more about this method (Lasater et al., 2015). The GRADE system is used by more than 100 organizations representing 19 countries worldwide. Its international organization members include the Cochrane Collaboration and World Health Organization. Among its US membership includes the Agency for Healthcare Research and Quality (AHRQ) and Institute for Clinical Improvement (Wang et al., 2016).

In the US, a variety of methods are employed and, different from NICE guidelines, an economic evaluation of the intervention or preventive service is not conducted. The U.S. Preventive Services Task Force (USPSTF), an independent group entrusted with creating guidelines about a broad range of clinical preventive services for adults and children, grades evidence for its recommendations from High, where the evidence is unlikely to be affected by results of future studies, to Low, where evidence is insufficient to make a recommendation; recommendations for practice range from encouraging routine use (Grade A) to discouraging use (Grade D). When evidence is either lacking, conflicting, or of poor quality, the recommendation is graded as I (insufficient evidence to recommend) (Goudreau et al., 2015). The USPSTF publishes its *Guide to Clinical Prevention Services* (Kumar et al., 2015), which summarizes key recommendations from more than 80 guidelines developed by the USPSTF. Although nurses may serve as members of guideline committees, they are often underutilized in this role.

In the US, national clinical organizations, trade organizations, and hospitals/health systems often fill the role of guideline developer within their specific expertise domain. Guideline recommendations often differ by guideline. For example, among the six clinical practice guidelines for hemoglobin A1c targets for adults with type 2 diabetes reviewed by Qaseem et al. (Qaseem et al., 2018), four of the six guidelines were developed in the US (one national clinical organization, two trade organizations, and one health system organization). Not surprisingly, both the overall quality of each guideline, rating of evidence from studies that supported the recommendation, as well as its target A1c recommendations varied.

Table 8.3 compares the systems employed by SIGN and USPSTF to rate guideline evidence. Clearly defined in the SIGN evidence rating system is incorporation of risk of bias assessment of included evidence to either elevate or lower the evidence rating and strength of recommendation. Clearly defined in the USPSTF system is that the evidence to support a USPSTF

TABLE 8.3 ■ Comparison of SIGN and USPSTF Evidence Rating Systems

SIGN		USPSTF	
Level of Evidence			
Level	*Determination*	*Grade*	*Determination*
1++	High-quality meta-analyses or systematic reviews of RCT with low risk of bias	High	Evidence includes results from studies with low risk of bias conducted in representative primary care samples; unlikely to be affected by results of future studies
1	Meta-analyses, systematic review of RCTs, or individual RCT; 1+ if low risk of bias; 1– if high risk of bias		
2++	High-quality systematic reviews of observational studies with low risk of bias and likely to establish causal relationship	Moderate	Evidence sufficient to determine effect of service on health outcomes, but estimate constrained and future studies could change observed effect
2	Well-conducted observational studies; 2+ if low risk of bias and moderate probability of establishing causality; 2– if high risk of bias and risk that relationship is not causal	Low	Evidence insufficient to assess health outcome effects
3	Case reports, case series		
4	Expert opinion		
Degree of Certainty			
Grade	*Determination*	*Level*	*Determination*
A	1++ evidence directly applicable to guideline target population OR majority 1+ evidence with consistent findings	A	Service recommended; high probability that net benefit is substantial
B	2++ body of evidence with consistent findings directly applicable to guideline target population OR extrapolated from 1++ or 1+ studies	B	Service recommended; high certainty that net benefit is moderate to substantial
C	2+ body of evidence with consistent findings directly applicable to guideline target population OR extrapolated from 2++ studies	C	Offer service selectively. At least moderate certainty that net benefit is small
D	3 or 4 evidence OR extrapolated from 2+ studies	D	Recommends against this service. Moderate or high certainty that service either has no net benefit or that harms outweigh benefits
		I	Evidence insufficient to assess service benefits and harms

RCT, Randomized controlled trial; *SIGN,* Scottish Intercollegiate Guidelines Network; *SR,* systematic review; *USPSTF,* U.S. Preventive Services Task Force.

guideline should stem from research conducted in representative primary care samples. However, how risk of bias is incorporated into evidence ratings for guidelines developed by USPSTF is less certain.

Integrating Guidelines into Clinical Practice

Although guidelines provide recommendations for best practice, they generally do not provide guidance regarding how to achieve change in practitioner behavior required for successful guideline implementation. Several evidence-based practice models are available to guide the implementation of guidelines into clinical practice settings (Schaffer et al., 2013). Here we briefly discuss three models: Knowledge to Action, Promoting Action on Research Implementation in Health Services (PARIHS), and Iowa models (for further description of these models and other frameworks, see Rycroft-Malone, J., Bucknall T. [Eds.], 2010. *Models and Frameworks for Implementing Evidence-Based Practice: Linking Evidence to Action.* Oxford: Wiley Blackwell).

The Knowledge to Action (KTA) model focuses on knowledge translation, a process that addresses the gap that lies between knowledge creation (research) and its implementation or translation into everyday practice (Field et al., 2014; Graham et al., 2006). In this model, knowledge creation (research) is at the center of the process (Fig. 8.1A). Once a practice problem has been identified and a guideline has been identified and appraised, a formal process for tailoring or adapting that knowledge to the local practice context is conducted. In addition, you need to identify potential barriers and/or facilitators to using the guideline so that all stakeholders affected by the practice change can be actively involved in the plan for change (intervention). After intervention implementation, how knowledge is used is monitored, and outcomes of the process are evaluated. Results are shared with stakeholders to support either further improvement or to sustain the change in practice.

The PARIHS model, first developed by Kitson, posits that successful implementation of knowledge into practices is reliant on three key elements: the nature of the evidence, the context into which it will be integrated, and how the change process is facilitated (Kitson et al., 1998). Just as identification of best evidence is critical, equal attention and importance must be given to preparing the local context for change and identifying the best facilitation method to optimize guideline uptake. If one element is lacking, implementation strategies will not be successful. Represented as a three-dimensional matrix, Fig. 8.1B illustrates the interplay between evidence, context, and facilitation. Implementation has the greatest probability of success when all elements are uniformly high. Effective facilitators possess and utilize a broad range of skills in project management and improvement, team building, negotiation, and influencing stakeholders for successful implementation to occur (Harvey and Kitson, 2016).

The Iowa Model, which has been recently revised based on experiences using the model and survey responses from 379 Iowa model users, is illustrated in Fig. 8.1C (Iowa Model Collaborative et al., 2017). In this model, the impetus for need for change in practice is identified through a trigger identified either locally (patient or clinician, institutional, or philosophy of care initiative) or new compelling evidence. Explicit in this model is that practice change has the highest chance of success when considered an institutional priority and when the evidence is sufficient to support the change. Once this is determined, the next steps are to develop and implement the plan, monitor change through data collection, and evaluate practice outcomes over time. Magnet hospitals in the US often employ the revised Iowa Model for implementation of evidence-based practice projects.

Although each implementation model contains unique qualities, some consistencies are evident across models. Each model has been widely used and stood the test of time. Espousers of each model acknowledge the complex nature of both the efforts needed to change behavior within

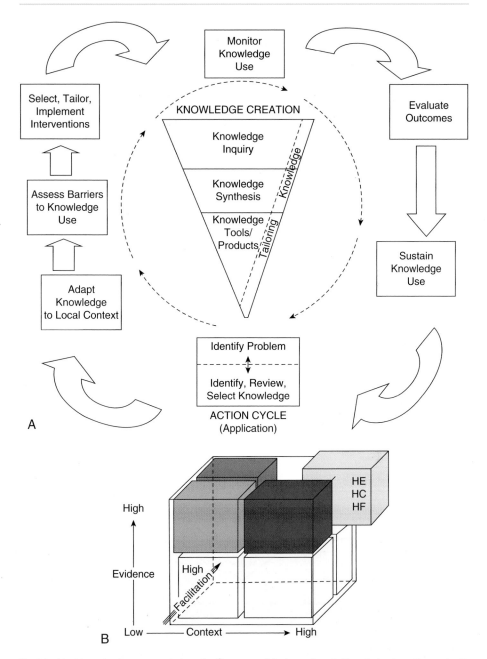

Fig. 8.1 Models to implement translation of evidence to clinical practice. A, Knowledge to action cycle. B, PARIHS Model; interplay between evidence, context, and facilitation. C, Iowa Model–Revised. (A, with permission from Graham, I.D., Logan, J., Harrison, M.B., Straus, S.E., Tetroe, J., Caswell, W., et al., 2006. Lost in knowledge translation: time for a map? J. Contin. Educ. Health Prof. 26 [1], 13–24. doi:10.1002/chp.47; B, with permission from Kitson, A., Harvey, G., McCormack, B., 1998. Enabling the implementation of evidence based practice: a conceptual framework. Qual. Health Care 7 [3], 149–158; C, with permission from Iowa Model Collaborative, Buckwalter, K.C., Cullen, L., Hanrahan, K., Kleiber, C., McCarthy, A.M.; Authored on behalf of the Iowa Model Collaborative, 2017. Iowa model of evidence-based practice: revisions and validation. Worldviews Evid. Based Nurs. 14 [3], 175–182. https://doi.org/10.1111/wvn.12223.)

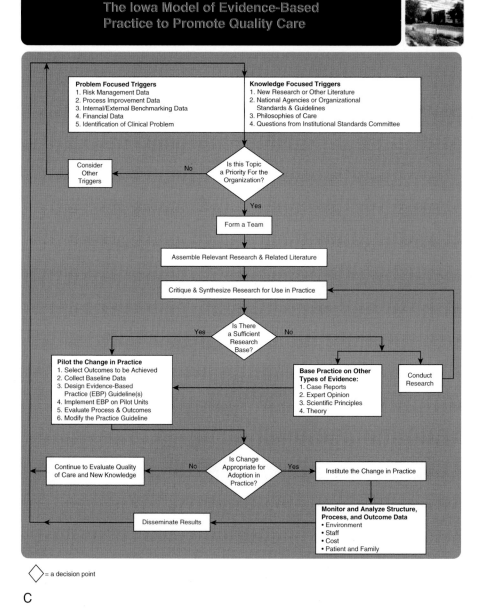

The Iowa Model of Evidence-Based Practice to Promote Quality Care

Problem Focused Triggers
1. Risk Management Data
2. Process Improvement Data
3. Internal/External Benchmarking Data
4. Financial Data
5. Identification of Clinical Problem

Knowledge Focused Triggers
1. New Research or Other Literature
2. National Agencies or Organizational Standards & Guidelines
3. Philosophies of Care
4. Questions from Institutional Standards Committee

Is this Topic a Priority For the Organization?

No → Consider Other Triggers

Yes

Form a Team

Assemble Relevant Research & Related Literature

Critique & Synthesize Research for Use in Practice

Is There a Sufficient Research Base?

Yes / No

Pilot the Change in Practice
1. Select Outcomes to be Achieved
2. Collect Baseline Data
3. Design Evidence-Based Practice (EBP) Guideline(s)
4. Implement EBP on Pilot Units
5. Evaluate Process & Outcomes
6. Modify the Practice Guideline

Base Practice on Other Types of Evidence:
1. Case Reports
2. Expert Opinion
3. Scientific Principles
4. Theory

Conduct Research

Is Change Appropriate for Adoption in Practice?

No → Continue to Evaluate Quality of Care and New Knowledge

Yes → Institute the Change in Practice

Monitor and Analyze Structure, Process, and Outcome Data
• Environment
• Staff
• Cost
• Patient and Family

Disseminate Results

◇ = a decision point

C

Fig. 8.1, cont'd

organizational settings and level of resources required to be successful. Therefore the evidence level supporting the need for practice change must be both compelling and viewed as an organizational priority. Identification of potential barriers to successful implementation is part of each model: this step is explicit in the KTA model but more implicit in the PARIHS and Iowa models. All models require champions to assure successful implementation and an evaluation phase to examine outcomes and their sustainability over time.

Conclusions

Use of clinical guidelines is inherent to clinical practice that is safe and reflects best evidence. As the largest component of the healthcare workforce, active engagement by nurses in both the development and implementation of guidelines is critical. Nurses will be involved with guideline implementation in a variety of ways: by identifying practice problems where change in practice is needed, identifying best evidence from guidelines to support that change, and either leading or serving on implementation teams to promote and sustain practice change. Each of these roles require prerequisite competency in the fundamental skills of identifying, appraising, and examining the level of evidence on which recommendations are based. After identification of best evidence, three widely employed implementation models are recommended to promote the successful translation of evidence to practice.

Opportunities for Further Education

There are a number of resources that you can use to get more information and access education about both the process of developing and implementing clinical guidelines. Each organization mentioned in this chapter provides access to resources on its website. In addition, the Joanna Briggs Institute (JBI) and the Guideline International Network (GIN) organize conferences and other continuing educational opportunities that may be of interest to nurses aspiring to taking greater leadership roles in evidence-based practice activities at their institutions.

First established at the University of Adelaide, Australia, the JBI has developed a global footprint, with JBI centers located on each continent. Of these, ten centers are located in the US, with two specifically located within schools of nursing. JBI offers a wide array of educational offerings (http://joannabriggs.org/education/short-courses#online-courses) including systematic review and GRADE methodology as well as a 6-month evidence-based clinical fellowship program.

The GIN was founded in 2002; its multi-disciplinary membership includes individuals and organizations from 47 countries around the globe. GIN serves as a repository of more than 6000 regularly updated guideline documents that are available to its membership. GIN's goal is to improve healthcare quality through international cooperation in promoting systematic development and utilization of clinical guidelines. Membership is available to nurses. GIN provides a number of educational resources for its members and the public. Recordings and slide sets from recent webinars are available at https://www.g-i-n.net/library/webinars/g-i-n-n-a-webinars.

References

Baird, A.G., Lawrence, J.R., 2014. Guidelines: is bigger better? A review of SIGN guidelines. BMJ Open 4 (2), e004278. https://doi.org/10.1136/bmjopen-2013-004278.

Bhaumik, S., 2017. Use of evidence for clinical practice guideline development. Trop. Parasitol. 7 (2), 65–71. https://doi.org/10.4103/tp.TP_6_17.

Brouwers, M.C., Kho, M.E., Browman, G.P., Burgers, J.S., Cluzeau, F., Feder, G., AGREE Next Steps Consortium, 2010. AGREE II: advancing guideline development, reporting, and evaluation in health care. Prev. Med. 51 (5), 421–424. https://doi.org/10.1016/j.ypmed.2010.08.005.

Clark, E., Donovan, E.F., Schoettker, P., 2006. From outdated to updated, keeping clinical guidelines valid. Int. J. Qual. Health Care 18 (3), 165–166. https://doi.org/10.1093/intqhc/mzl007.

Dahlqvist Jonsson, P., Schon, U.K., Rosenberg, D., Sandlund, M., Svedberg, P., 2015. Service users' experiences of participation in decision making in mental health services. J. Psychiatr. Mental Health Nurs. 22 (9), 688–697. https://dx.doi.org/10.1111/jpm.12246.

Dijkers, M., 2013. Introducing GRADE: a systematic approach to rating evidence in systematic reviews and to guideline development. KT Update 1 (5). Available from: ktdrr.org/products/update/v1n5/dijkers_grade_ktupdatev1n5.pdf (Accessed 03.05.19).

Duda, S., Fahim, C., Szatmari, P., Bennett, K., 2017. Is the National Guideline Clearinghouse a trustworthy source of practice guidelines for child and youth anxiety and depression? J. Can. Acad. Child Adolesc. Psychiatry 26 (2), 86–97.

Ebben, R.H., Vloet, L.C., van Grunsven, P.M., Breeman, W., Goosselink, B., Lichtveld, R.A., et al., 2015. Factors influencing ambulance nurses' adherence to a national protocol ambulance care: an implementation study in the Netherlands. Eur. J. Emerg. Med. 22 (3), 199–205. https://doi.org/10.1097/MEJ.0000000000000133.

Field, B., Booth, A., Ilott, I., Gerrish, K., 2014. Using the knowledge to action framework in practice: a citation analysis and systematic review. Implement. Sci. 9, 172. https://doi.org/10.1186/s13012-014-0172-2.

Forberg, U., Wallin, L., Johansson, E., Ygge, B.M., Backheden, M., Ehrenberg, A., 2014. Relationship between work context and adherence to a clinical practice guideline for peripheral venous catheters among registered nurses in pediatric care. Worldviews Evid. Based Nurs. 11 (4), 227–239. https://doi.org/10.1111/wvn.12046.

Fuentes Padilla, P., Martinez, G., Vernooij, R.W.M., Cosp, X.B., Alonso-Coello, P., 2016. Nutrition in critically ill adults: a systematic quality assessment of clinical practice guidelines. Clin. Nutr. 35 (6), 1219–1225. https://doi.org/10.1016/j.clnu.2016.03.005.

Goudreau, J., Pepin, J., Larue, C., Dubois, S., Descoteaux, R., Lavoie, P., et al., 2015. A competency-based approach to nurses' continuing education for clinical reasoning and leadership through reflective practice in a care situation. Nurse Educ. Pract. 15 (6), 572–578. https://dx.doi.org/10.1016/j.nepr.2015.10.013.

Graham, I.D., Logan, J., Harrison, M.B., Straus, S.E., Tetroe, J., Caswell, W., et al., 2006. Lost in knowledge translation: time for a map? J. Contin. Educ. Health Prof. 26 (1), 13–24. https://doi.org/10.1002/chp.47.

Handelsman, Y., Bloomgarden, Z.T., Grunberger, G., Umpierrez, G., Zimmerman, R.S., Bailey, T.S., et al., 2015. American Association of Clinical Endocrinologists and American College of Endocrinology clinical practice guidelines for developing a diabetes mellitus comprehensive care plan. Endocr. Pract. 21 (Suppl. 1), 1–87. https://doi.org/10.4158/EP15672.GL.

Harvey, G., Kitson, A., 2016. PARIHS revisited: from heuristic to integrated framework for the successful implementation of knowledge into practice. Implement. Sci. 11, 33. https://doi.org/10.1186/s13012-016-0398-2.

Hoffmann-Eßer, W., Siering, U., Neugebauer, E.A., Brockhaus, A.C., Lampert, U., Eikermann, M., 2017a. Guideline appraisal with AGREE II: systematic review of the current evidence on how users handle the 2 overall assessments. PLoS One 12 (3), e0174831. https://doi.org/10.1371/journal.pone.0174831.

Hoffmann-Eßer, W., Siering, U., Neugebauer, E.A.M., Lampert, U., Eikermann, M., 2018. Is there a cut-off for high-quality guidelines? A systematic analysis of current guideline appraisals using the AGREE II instrument. J. Clin. Epidemiol. 95, 120–127. https://doi.org/10.1016/j.jclinepi.2017.12.009.

Holmer, H.K., Ogden, L.A., Burda, B.U., Norris, S.L., 2013. Quality of clinical practice guidelines for glycemic control in type 2 diabetes mellitus. PLoS One 8 (4), e58625. https://doi.org/10.1371/journal.pone.0058625.

Graham, R., Mancher, M., Miller Wolman, D., Greenfield, S., Steinberg, E. (Eds.), 2011. Institute of Medicine (US) Committee on Standards for Developing Trustworthy Clinical Practice Guidelines. Clinical Practice Guidelines We Can Trust. National Academies Press, Washington, DC.

Iowa Model Collaborative, Buckwalter, K.C., Cullen, L., Hanrahan, K., Kleiber, C., McCarthy, A.M., Authored on behalf of the Iowa Model Collaborative, 2017. Iowa model of evidence-based practice: revisions and validation. Worldviews Evid. Based Nurs. 14 (3), 175–182. https://doi.org/10.1111/wvn.12223.

Jun, J., Kovner, C.T., Stimpfel, A.W., 2016. Barriers and facilitators of nurses' use of clinical practice guidelines: an integrative review. Int. J. Nurs. Stud. 60, 54–68. https://doi.org/10.1016/j.ijnurstu.2016.03.006.

Kitson, A., Harvey, G., McCormack, B., 1998. Enabling the implementation of evidence based practice: a conceptual framework. Qual. Health Care 7 (3), 149–158.

Kumar, K., Jones, D., Naden, K., Roberts, C., 2015. Rural and remote young people's health career decision making within a health workforce development program: a qualitative exploration. Rural Remote Health 15 (4), 3303.

Lasater, K., Nielsen, A.E., Stock, M., Ostrogorsky, T.L., 2015. Evaluating the clinical judgment of newly hired staff nurses. J. Contin. Educ. Nurs. 46 (12), 563–571. https://dx.doi.org/10.3928/00220124-20151112-09.

Lytvyn, L., Mertz, D., Sadeghirad, B., Alaklobi, F., Selva, A., Alonso-Coello, P., et al., 2016. Prevention of *Clostridium difficile* infection: a systematic survey of clinical practice guidelines. Infect. Control Hosp. Epidemiol. 37 (8), 901–908. https://doi.org/10.1017/ice.2016.104.

Martinez Garcia, L., Arevalo-Rodriguez, I., Sola, I., Haynes, R.B., Vandvik, P.O., Alonso-Coello, P., Updating Guidelines Working Group, 2012. Strategies for monitoring and updating clinical practice guidelines: a systematic review. Implement. Sci. 7, 109. https://doi.org/10.1186/1748-5908-7-109.

Maymone, M.B.C., Gan, S.D., Bigby, M., 2014. Evaluating the strength of clinical recommendations in the medical literature: GRADE, SORT, and AGREE. J. Invest. Dermatol. 134 (10), 1–5. https://doi.org/10.1038/jid.2014.335.

National Guideline Clearinghouse, 2012. Fact sheet, 2012. Available from: https://www.nice.org.uk/process/pmg20/chapter/introduction-and-overview#information-about-this-manual (Accessed 03.05.19).

National Institute for Health and Care Excellence (NICE), 2014. Developing NICE guidelines: the manual. Available from: https://www.nice.org.uk/process/pmg20/chapter/introduction-and-overview#information-about-this-manual (Accessed 03.05.19).

National Institute for Health and Care Excellence (NICE), 2018. Improving health and social care through evidence-based guidance, 2018. Available from: https://www.nice.org.uk (Accessed 03.05.19).

Neuman, M.D., Goldstein, J.N., Cirullo, M.A., Schwartz, J.S., 2014. Durability of class I American College of Cardiology/American Heart Association clinical practice guideline recommendations. JAMA 311 (20), 2092–2100. https://doi.org/10.1001/jama.2014.4949.

Qaseem, A., Forland, F., Macbeth, F., Ollenschlager, G., Phillips, S., van der Wees, P., Board of Trustees of the Guidelines International, Network, 2012. Guidelines International Network: toward international standards for clinical practice guidelines. Ann. Intern. Med. 156 (7), 525–531. https://doi.org/10.7326/0003-4819-156-7-201204030-00009.

Qaseem, A., Wilt, T.J., Kansagara, D., Horwitch, C., Barry, M.J., Forciea, M.A., Clinical Guidelines Committee of the American College of Physicians, 2018. Hemoglobin A1c targets for glycemic control with pharmacologic therapy for nonpregnant adults with type 2 diabetes mellitus: a guidance statement update from the American College of Physicians. Ann. Intern. Med. 168 (8), 569–576. https://doi.org/10.7326/M17-0939.

Ransohoff, D.F., Sox, H.C., 2013. Guidelines for guidelines: measuring trustworthiness. J. Clin. Oncol. 31 (20), 2530–2531. https://doi.org/10.1200/JCO.2013.50.0462.

Schaffer, M.A., Sandau, K.E., Diedrick, L., 2013. Evidence-based practice models for organizational change: overview and practical applications. J. Adv. Nurs. 69 (5), 1197–1209. https://doi.org/10.1111/j.1365-2648.2012.06122.x.

Schneider, E.C., Sarnak, D.O., Squires, D., Shah, A., Doty, M.M., 2017. Mirror, mirror 2017: International comparison reflects flaws and opportunities for better U.S. health care. Available from: http://www.commonwealthfund.org/interactives/2017/july/mirror-mirror/assets/Schneider_mirror_mirror_2017.pdf (Accessed 03.05.19).

Shaku, F., Tsutsumi, M., 2016. The effect of providing life support on nurses' decision making regarding life support for themselves and family members in Japan. Am. J. Hospice Palliat. Med. 33 (10), 917–923. https://dx.doi.org/10.1177/1049909115624655.

Shekelle, P., Woolf, S., Grimshaw, J.M., Schunemann, H.J., Eccles, M.P., 2012. Developing clinical practice guidelines: reviewing, reporting, and publishing guidelines; updating guidelines; and the emerging issues of enhancing guideline implementability and accounting for comorbid conditions in guideline development. Implement. Sci. 7, 62. https://doi.org/10.1186/1748-5908-7-62.

Shekelle, P.G., Ortiz, E., Rhodes, S., Morton, S.C., Eccles, M.P., Grimshaw, J.M., et al., 2001. Validity of the Agency for Healthcare Research and Quality clinical practice guidelines: how quickly do guidelines become outdated? JAMA 286 (12), 1461–1467.

Siering, U., Eikermann, M., Hausner, E., Hoffmann-Esser, W., Neugebauer, E.A., 2013. Appraisal tools for clinical practice guidelines: a systematic review. PLoS One 8 (12), e82915. https://doi.org/10.1371/journal.pone.0082915.

Thornton, J., Alderson, P., Tan, T., Turner, C., Latchem, S., Shaw, E., et al., 2013. Introducing GRADE across the NICE clinical guideline program. J. Clin. Epidemiol. 66 (2), 124–131. https://doi.org/10.1016/j.jclinepi.2011.12.007.

Uhlig, K., Berns, J.S., Carville, S., Chan, W., Cheung, M., Guyatt, G.H., et al., 2016. Recommendations for kidney disease guideline updating: a report by the KDIGO Methods Committee. Kidney Int. 89 (4), 753–760. https://doi.org/10.1016/j.kint.2015.11.030.

Vernooij, R.W., Sanabria, A.J., Sola, I., Alonso-Coello, P., Martinez Garcia, L., 2014. Guidance for updating clinical practice guidelines: a systematic review of methodological handbooks. Implement. Sci. 9, 3. https://doi.org/10.1186/1748-5908-9-3.

Wang, L.H., Goopy, S., Lin, C.C., Barnard, A., Han, C.Y., Liu, H.E., 2016. The emergency patient's participation in medical decision-making. J. Clin. Nurs. 25 (17-18), 2550–2558. https://dx.doi.org/10.1111/jocn.13296.

CHAPTER 9

Using Research Evidence in Making Clinical Decisions with Individual Patients

Dawn Dowding

KEY POINTS

- Evidence from high-quality research studies should form the basis for making clinical decisions with and for individual patients.
- Techniques such as Bayesian probability revision and decision analysis are useful tools to assist with making clinical decisions for individual patients.
- An evidence-based decision should incorporate patient values and their preferences for different treatments or outcomes.
- Be aware that how we communicate information to patients can affect the decisions they make.
- How individuals understand risks and benefits differs. Consider communicating the same information in different ways.
- Decision support tools and decision aids can help incorporate evidence into clinical decisions.

Introduction

A number of terms, such as "clinical reasoning," "clinical judgment," "decision-making," and "diagnostic reasoning" are often used to describe the same phenomenon (Simmons, 2010): using information to make judgments (evaluations) and decisions (choices) about a patient's condition. In an evidence-based approach to patient care, the information should be the highest-quality research evidence we can access. However, research evidence is not the only component of evidence-informed decision-making; a patient's preferences for different treatments or outcomes and the availability (or lack thereof) of funds, resources, and clinical skill/expertise to provide a particular intervention are also important components in the decision process (Yost et al., 2014, 2015). Furthermore, making clinical decisions with individual patients involves not just considering the implications of the evidence for that patient, but also helping them to apply it to their own individual circumstances.

One of the challenges of evidence-based practice is that of knowing how to take the research evidence generated by studying samples of patients and applying it to the decisions made with individual patients. This chapter examines practical ways in which you can do this and discusses approaches that you can use to help patients to understand the evidence, to assist them with their decision-making. It also considers how you can take into account patients' views or preferences about their treatment, and the role of shared decision-making in evidence-based practice.

By necessity, the discussion of strategies for applying evidence to decision-making for individual patients, derived from decision-making research and teaching, is brief. Interested readers are directed to the further reading at the end of this chapter.

Does the Evidence Fit?

One of the first challenges in using evidence to help with decisions in practice is establishing that the research evidence is appropriate for the situation you are faced with. Examples of the different types of judgments and decisions taken by nurses in practice, which have been developed from seminal studies exploring nurses' judgments and decision-making in both primary and acute care (Lamond et al., 1996; Thompson et al. 2001, 2004), can be seen in Table 9.1. They include diagnostic judgments (assessments) as well as decisions related to what interventions to choose and the timing and targeting of such interventions.

TABLE 9.1 ■ Types of Judgements and Decisions, and Examples of What They Look Like in Practice

Types of Judgments/Decisions	Clinical Examples
Diagnostic/evaluative (the cause of a problem/a patient's health status)	• Nurse diagnoses the cause of a patient's incontinence (based on information collected during a full assessment) • Nurse judges the patient is "stable" (based on information collected during an assessment)
Prognostic (the likely future outcome/ the course of a disease)	• Nurse judges that the patient will have problems postoperatively (based on information collected about the patient preoperatively) • Nurse chooses what information to communicate to an elderly patient who has had a myocardial infarction, and her relatives who are worrying about her chances of having another heart attack
Treatment (the most effective intervention/the best timing to deploy the intervention/the type of service that is most appropriate to deliver the intervention)	• Nurse chooses a mattress for a frail elderly man who has been admitted with an acute bowel obstruction • Nurse chooses which management strategy is likely to prevent recurrence of a healed leg ulcer • Nurse chooses a time to begin asthma education for a newly diagnosed patient with asthma • Nurse decides which patients should receive antiembolic stockings • Nurse chooses that a patient's leg ulcer is arterial rather than venous and so merits medical rather than nursing management in the community • Nurse chooses how to organize handover so that communication is most effective (in this example, handover can be thought of as an intervention or "treatment")
Patient's needs	• Nurse chooses how to reassure a patient who is worried about cardiac arrest after witnessing another patient arresting

(Modified from Thompson, C., Aitken, L., Doran, D., Dowding, D., 2013. An agenda for clinical decision making and judgment in nursing research and education. Int. J. Nurs. Stud. 50 [12], 1720–1726.)

What this typology illustrates is that you are likely to be faced with a diversity of judgments and decisions in your everyday clinical practice and, consequently, a number of different types of questions for which you will need answers. There is a direct link between the decision problem you are faced with, the type of clinical question you are asking, and the type of research study design needed to help you answer the question and subsequently make your decision. A clinical scenario illustrates this linkage (Box 9.1). The point here is that if you can identify what type of decision you are making, it may help you to focus both your question and your search of the relevant literature.

As discussed in previous chapters, once you have identified relevant research evidence, you will need to reassure yourself of its validity and determine its usefulness for your individual patient. The latter involves assessing the similarity of (i) the context of the research study and your particular clinical environment, (ii) the patient group investigated in the study and the particular clinical circumstances of your patient, and (iii) the application of the intervention/investigation under study conditions and the intervention/investigation that you plan to provide in your setting. At the end of this process, if you have determined that the research evidence is relevant to your particular decision scenario, you still have to try and incorporate it into your decision-making for this individual patient.

Strategies for Decision-Making

The majority of studies examining how nurses make decisions in practice suggest that they use a variety of different types of reasoning including hypothetico-deductive reasoning (e.g., Jefford et al., 2011), heuristics and biases (e.g., Patterson et al., 2015), and intuition (e.g., Gillespie et al., 2015), depending on the clinical context and their own expertise. A brief description of each approach is given in Box 9.2. However, what characterizes these types of reasoning is the lack of any distinction between research evidence (i.e., the experiences of hundreds or even thousands of patients) and other kinds of evidence (such as a sense of intuitive "correctness" in the course of action you are considering) as a basis for formulating decisions. Ignoring research (where it exists and is suitable) can lead to systematic errors or biases in reasoning and poor decision-making in practice.

The rest of this section explores approaches to decision-making that enable you explicitly to include research evidence in the decision process. These techniques are not all designed for scenarios in which you need to make a decision quickly. However, if you have taken the time to ask a question, search for evidence, and appraise the evidence, it is worth expending the additional time to consider how to use the evidence effectively for your individual patient.

BOX 9.1 ■ The Link Between Decisions, Questions, and Study Designs

Mr. Smith, a 35-year-old man with a history of smoking, visits your primary care practice for a follow-up consultation after a chest infection. You advise him that he probably should try to stop smoking and discuss his treatment options with him. A number of options are available to him, including the use of various types of nicotine replacement therapy and counseling programs (both face-to-face and on the Internet). He wants to know whether using an online resource would be as effective in helping him to stop smoking as some sort of face-to-face support (either individually or in a group) as he travels a lot and would find it difficult to keep a number of face-to-face appointments.

Type of decision: Intervention: involves choosing among alternatives
Type of clinical question: Effectiveness of a treatment
Type of study design: The optimum study design for a question about the effectiveness of a treatment is a systematic review of randomized controlled trials (RCTs) or an RCT.

BOX 9.2 ■ Types of Clinical Reasoning (Based on Theories of How People Actually—Rather Than Ought to—Make Decisions)

Information Processing

Decision makers as active information seekers (or at least receivers of information), able to synthesize the information they are exposed to and make sense of it. A common mistake is to view reasoning as being "like a computer"; [unlike a computer] decision makers have their processing "bounded" (Marwala and Hurwitz, 2017) by limited processing power, imperfect information, time constraints, and other external factors.

Hypothetico-Deductive Reasoning

Decision makers reason using stages. Perhaps the most well known being (Elstein et al. 1978) proposal that clinical reasoning consists of four key stages: (a) cue acquisition in which clinical information is gathered, (b) hypothesis generation in which the clinician formulates ideas about what might be happening, (c) cue interpretation in which the meaning of the cues *given* the working hypotheses is established, and (d) hypothesis evaluation in which the ideas of what might be happening are tested and either rejected or more information gathered.

Intuitive Judgment and Decision-Making

This is a very attractive label for nurse theorists and scholars. Intuition is itself contested, but commonly refers to variations of "knowing without knowing quite why you know." As knowledge, intuition is largely invisible and impossible to share with others (how can you share something when you do not know what it is you are sharing?). As a way of knowing, intuition is likely to draw on cognitive shortcuts (see later) called "heuristics" and the systematic errors that can result. Intuition can be a powerful tool in the hands of experts (e.g., see the seminal work of Benner and Tanner, 1987; Benner, 1984).

Heuristics (and their Biases)

Decision makers rely on "shortcuts" to handle complex information in decisions, and this can result in predictable errors. By way of explanation, a person who is overconfident in the correctness of his or her knowledge, for example in his or her correctness in estimating risk, may have a false confidence in his or her ability to make accurate judgments and, as a result, may act inappropriately; the person may fail to act when urgent action is required to mitigate the risk or may be overzealous in his or her actions (Yang et al., 2012). Heuristic-based reasoning is often portrayed as a negative phenomena; however, they can also be an effective way to make decisions in time-constrained situations (Gigerenzer and Gaissmaier, 2011).

The Cognitive Continuum

In this approach, the reasoning style you employ is neither wholly rational nor wholly intuitive. Rather, the problem you are faced with determines (in part) the style of reasoning you employ (so a decision with no time constraints might be made using decision analysis, but the same decision with no time available will lead to intuitive reasoning).

Dual-Processing Theory (System I and System II Thinking)

This is the concept that we use different types of cognitive processing, depending on the situation and time available. System I thinking is characterized by fast, intuitive type thinking, and System II is characterized by slower and more deliberative thought. Although System I is generally considered to be our default approach to decision-making, it can lead to bias; with a suggestion we should be focusing on using more System II deliberative thinking (Evans, 2011; Kahneman, 2013).

USING EVIDENCE IN DIAGNOSTIC DECISION-MAKING

The process of diagnosis involves using the information we have collected about a patient's medical history, test results, signs, and symptoms to try and identify what the cause of her or his current complaint may be (Thompson and Dowding, 2009). Research evidence can provide information about the likelihood that an individual has a particular disease, as well as providing data on how

---

BOX 9.3 ■ Using Evidence in Diagnosis

You are a primary care nurse practitioner. A 51-year-old woman who is attending clinic for her cervical smear test tells you that she had a mammogram 2 weeks ago. The test result has come back as "suspicious," and she has been told that she now needs to go to the hospital for further tests. She asks you if this means she has cancer.

What is the Likelihood that a 51-Year-Old Woman has Breast Cancer?

The incidence rate for breast cancer in women 50 to 64 years of age (latest statistics available from 2014) in the US (all races) is 263.65 per 100,000 population) (North American Association of Central Cancer Registries, 2018).

How Good is a Mammogram at Detecting Cancer in 51-Year-Old Women?

Mammography has a sensitivity (chances of the test being positive, given that the patient has the condition) of between 77% and 95%, and a specificity (chances of the test being negative, given that the patient does not have the disease) of 94% to 97% (Siu and USPSTF, 2016).

---

accurate a diagnostic test is within a particular patient population. This section focuses on an approach, known as Bayes' rule. Bayes theorem a set of rules for making sense of uncertain information in diagnostic decisions.

Bayes' rule or theorem can be described as:

The likelihood of patient X having a disease or condition (posterior probability)
= the likelihood of patient X having disease or condition before you collected any evidence (prior probability)
× the strength of the evidence you have collected

Look at the example given in Box 9.3. To answer this woman's question, you would need to know:

■ how likely it is that a 51-year-old woman has breast cancer (prior probability)
■ the performance or accuracy of mammograms for identifying breast cancer in 51-year-old women (strength of evidence)

With this information, you can then calculate what the likelihood is that the woman does actually have breast cancer (posterior probability). Before we look at the evidence, write down what you think the chances are that the woman has breast cancer, given your knowledge and experience.

Your learning from the previous chapters should stand you in good stead to identify the evidence needed to answer this question. You need to use the PICO (population, intervention, comparison, outcome) approach to focus your question, search for the appropriate evidence, and then try to specifically answer the woman's question. The evidence identified for the purposes of this example is summarized in Box 9.3.

You now have the components needed in Bayes' rule to calculate the likelihood or chance that, given a positive test result, your patient does actually have cancer. One of the easiest ways to do this is to use an online calculator such as the one found online at: http://araw.mede.uic.edu/cgi-bin/testcalc.pl. You enter the prevalence of the disease condition (prior probability), which in this case is 263.7/100,000 or 0.003. You also enter the sensitivity (0.77–0.95) and specificity (0.94–0.97). To obtain the full range of confidence intervals, first enter the lower values for sensitivity and specificity and calculate, then the higher set of values. Given this information, the probability or likelihood of the woman having breast cancer (posterior probability) is calculated. The results of this are displayed in a number of ways, with data on what the results of a positive test mean, and data on what a negative test mean displayed separately. Depending on how accurate the mammography screening is (i.e., how good it is at detecting both positive and negative cases), the woman's probability (the posterior probability for a positive test) of having breast cancer has risen to between 4% and 9%.

What this also indicates is the number of women who are "false positives," in other words the number of women who have a positive test result despite not having the disease. The estimates for this particular test indicate between 1 in 11 and 1 in 27 women who have a positive mammogram actually have breast cancer (i.e., between 10 in 11 or 26 in 27 women who have a positive mammogram DO NOT have breast cancer). So, even though the woman described in Box 9.3 has had a positive test and her chances of having breast cancer have increased, it is still more likely that it is a false alarm.

Using Bayes' rule can help you evaluate how useful the signs and symptoms of particular diseases are for deciding if a patient has a given condition/disease; it helps determine the utility of diagnostic test results in particular groups of patients. It can also help you determine whether or not it is worthwhile to carry out a particular test for an individual patient. If the new information will not provide a greater insight into whether or not the patient either has or does not have the disease, it may not be worthwhile conducting the test. In instances such as the one described in Box 9.3, where there is a high chance of a false-positive test result, it may be worth discussing both the benefits and limitations of the test with the patient. The worry and additional testing associated with testing positive, for some patients, may outweigh the potential benefits provided by the test.

USING EVIDENCE IN TREATMENT DECISION-MAKING

When we are discussing treatment decision-making, we are normally trying to decide which of a number of options (including doing nothing or "watchful waiting") is the best approach for the patient, hopefully in collaboration with the patient. Research evidence can provide us with information about the comparative effectiveness of the different alternatives available, as well as their possible adverse or side effects. Often in health care, there is no one "obvious" alternative that is better than the others, perhaps due to the tradeoffs in terms of risks and benefits. The preferences and views of the individual patient are thus particularly important for helping inform what the best course of action may be. In these circumstances, a more formal approach to decision-making, such as decision analysis, can help.

We will not guide you through the entire process of carrying out a decision analysis in this text (both Hunink et al., 2014 and Dowding and Thompson, 2009 provide a more detailed guide), but we do need to visit the principles of the approach. Decision analysis uses decision trees to structure the decision problem being faced, incorporates information from research evidence (in the form of probabilities or likelihood of certain events occurring) to the branches of the trees, and combines these with a formal evaluation of the patient's values or preferences (known as utility) for different outcomes, to reach an optimum decision.

To illustrate these principles, we use the example of a woman suffering from menopausal symptoms who needs to make a treatment decision.

In this example, the main clinical problem experienced by the woman is the hot flashes associated with menopause. The woman has been advised that having a healthy lifestyle (regular exercise, a heart-healthy diet, no smoking, and limiting caffeine, alcohol, and stress) as well as hormone therapy (HT) (estrogen only) may help alleviate these symptoms. Possible outcomes of these interventions include: improvement or no improvement of hot flashes, increased risks of stroke and venous thromboembolism, and reduced risks of coronary events, fractures, and breast cancer (Marjoribanks et al., 2017). This example focuses on breast cancer, but any (or all) of the potential outcomes of taking HT could be included in the decision model.

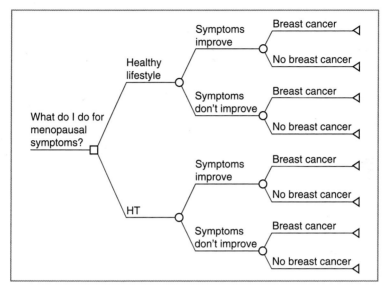

Fig. 9.1 Structure of a decision tree.

A decision tree helps to graphically display this information. As shown in Fig. 9.1, the tree is easy to draw and should include: the problem (always shown to the left of the tree); the decision choices (represented by a square node), that is, healthy lifestyle alone (comprising regular exercise and a healthy diet) or the addition of HT; and the possible "chance" outcomes for each decision (represented by circle nodes), that is, hot flashes improve or do not improve. For each of these chance branches, there are two further possible chance outcomes: development of breast cancer or no breast cancer. The chances of other outcomes occurring are not shown on the tree, but could easily be added.

Next, the probability of each of these outcomes occurring needs to be added to each branch of the tree, as shown in Fig. 9.2. Where it is available, high-quality research evidence, adapted for the individual patient's prognostic factors, can be used to give the probability or likelihood of certain events occurring (for this example, data have been taken from systematic reviews by Daley et al., 2014, Marjoribanks et al., 2017, and MacLennan et al., 2004). In the absence of research data, other estimations of likelihood (such as expert estimation) can be used, on the understanding that this type of evidence is less reliable than that derived from research. One of the key characteristics of research-derived probabilities is that they vary in samples and the populations to which they are applied, so measures of variability, extracted from the published research, are often helpful in decision analysis. For example, confidence intervals for the probabilities can be used to construct upper and lower estimates for an individual and (later on in the process) the decision tested to see what happens to the optimal choice for an individual when the probabilities differ.

The final part of the decision tree entails evaluating patient's values, or utility, for the different outcomes (see the following section) and adding this information to the tree. Utilities are usually expressed as a number between 0 (worst possible health state) and 1 or 100 (best possible health state), as shown in Fig. 9.3. They are used as a measure of patient preference in the decision tree, and as such are a formal inclusion of patients' values into the decision process.

Once both probabilities and utilities are added into the tree, the best possible decision option is calculated. Probabilities and utilities for each decision branch are multiplied and then added

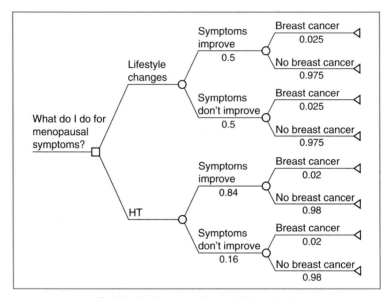

Fig. 9.2   Decision tree with probabilities added.

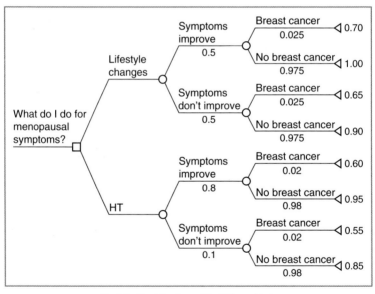

Fig. 9.3   Decision tree with utilities added.

together, until each decision option being considered has an overall number made up of the sum of all of its branches (Fig. 9.4). Here's how it is done:

Multiply the utility value for breast cancer at top right of tree (0.7) with the probability of that outcome (0.025) to yield 0.02.

For the branch below, multiply the utility value for no breast cancer (1.0) with the probability of that outcome (0.975) to yield 0.975.

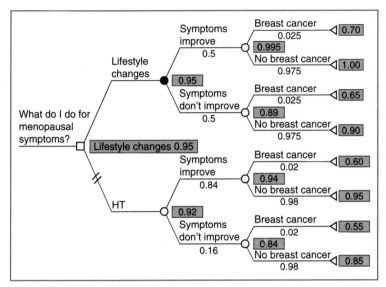

Fig. 9.4 Decision tree with full calculations.

Add the resultant figures together to yield the expected utility for *hot flashes improved:* 0.02 + 0.975 = 0.995.

Using the same formulas, carry out the calculations for the two branches of the chance node below to yield an expected utility for *hot flashes not improved:* 0.016 + 0.878 = 0.89.

Working back to the left of the tree, calculate the overall expected utility for lifestyle changes: (0.975 × 0.5) + (0.89 × 0.5) = 0.95.

Repeat this process to calculate the overall expected utility for HT: = 0.92

Decision analysis assumes that individuals are rational, logical decision makers who will choose the decision option most likely to result in an outcome that has the greatest utility for the individual (Marwala and Hurwitz, 2017). The decision option with the highest number is the one that maximizes an individual's expected utility, that is, is the option that is most likely to lead to an outcome that the individual decision maker values or prefers. In the decision tree in Fig. 9.4, the best option for this particular woman is to change her lifestyle (expected utility of 0.95).

If the same decision scenario were given to a woman who was not as severely affected by hot flashes associated with menopause and who therefore may have different values or utilities, this preferred option may change. The optimal decision may also change if the probability of different outcomes occurring was altered.

Decision analysis is not suitable for all healthcare decisions; it takes time and practice. But it can be a powerful tool for structuring decision problems, for formally ensuring that research evidence is incorporated into decisions about individual patients and that patient values are explicitly considered and taken account of.

Evaluating Patient Preferences

A key component of an evidence-based decision is ascertaining how a patient feels about the potential risks and benefits associated with different treatment options available to them. Approaches for exploring patients' preferences vary in formality and aims. "Value clarification exercises" are one way of helping patients clarify their own values to help them with a decision

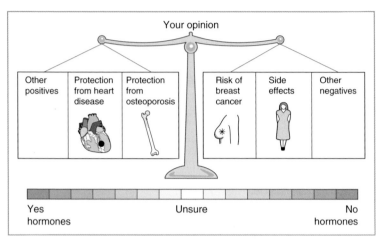

Fig. 9.5   An example of a values clarification exercise designed to help women participate in decisions regarding hormone replacement therapy. (From O'Connor, A., Wells, G., Tugwell, P., et al. 1999. The effects of an "explicit" values clarification exercise in a woman's decision aid regarding postmenopausal hormone therapy. Health Expect. 2 [1], 21–32, with permission.)

(Witteman et al., 2016). So, for example, a weigh scale, as shown in Fig. 9.5, may be used to help the individual identify and assign weight to the pros and cons of different treatment options; in this example to aid an informed choice about HT. Benefits and risks associated with the intervention are presented as "weights" on the scale, with benefits, or reasons to choose the intervention, shown on the left, and risks, or reasons to forego the intervention, shown on the right. The individual is asked to add any other reasons they can think of that may affect whether or not they would take HT. They are then asked to indicate how important each risk and benefit is to them by shading or assigning stars to each "weight" (completely shaded/5 stars = "very important to me"; through to no shading/no stars = "not at all important to me"). Having done this, they rate their predisposition toward taking HT on the scale underneath, which is anchored between taking and not taking HT, with being unsure in the middle (O'Connor et al., 1999). The exercises can be used by patients to guide their decision processes, and by healthcare professionals as a reference point for ensuring that they understand what is important to the patient.

A patient's valuation of an outcome or health state (i.e., the utility they assign to a particular outcome) is usually expressed on a scale ranging from "worst possible state of health" to "best possible state of health." As utility is an individual measure, it is possible that the worst and best possible health states will vary among individuals, as will their individual ratings of health states in between these two extremes. The simplest approach to formally assessing utility is to use a simple rating scale in which individuals are asked to rate outcomes on a scale from 0 (worst possible outcome) to 1 or 100 (best possible outcome). Other, more complex approaches include time trade-off techniques, and a standard gamble (for further explanation of these approaches see Dowding and Thompson, 2009).

Using utilities to measure patient preferences is not beyond criticism. The numbers associated with the utility for an outcome have been found to vary depending on the method used to generate them. Often, utility measures are carried out on a sample of individuals, and then assigned to an outcome within a decision analysis. These sample measures of utility may not be appropriate for individual patients, who may have different values and preferences to that represented by a group average, and it has been suggested that these approaches are not as robust as other methods of values clarification (Witteman et al., 2016). However, what does seem to be apparent is that methods that explicitly help people explore what matters to them and how that relates to the best treatment option for them may lead to more positive outcomes (Witteman et al., 2016).

Shared Decision-Making

Gathering utilities and probabilities only really makes sense if, as a clinician, you are committed to working with patients on the decisions that you both face. Aside from a general policy impetus (e.g., see the National Academy for State Health Policy report on Shared Decision Making) (Shafir and Rosenthal, 2012), there are also practical reasons why shared decision-making, defined as "when a health care provider and a patient work together to make a health care decision that works best for the patient" (Agency for Healthcare Research and Quality [AHRQ], 2014), helps. First, patients who are involved in their decisions are more knowledgeable and informed about their decisions, and they may make decisions more congruent with their values (Stacey et al., 2017). Second, the factors that we think are important in decision-making (quality-adjusted life years [QALYs], functional ability, pain) may not be the same factors that drive a patient's choice. For an example of how wrong we can be (researchers and clinicians), the OMERACT initiative in arthritis (http://www.ncbi.nlm.nih.gov/pmc/articles/PMC2169260/?tool=pubmed) arose directly from a recognition that the outcomes we measure in clinical trials of treatments of rheumatoid arthritis (pain, mobility) are not the same outcomes that matter to patients with rheumatoid arthritis (fatigue is the one most commonly cited). The third, and perhaps most compelling reason for an evidence-based clinician, is that patients all vary in their preferences (and, indeed, the probability of events/outcomes associated with choices). This variability begs the question: how will you know what your patient's preferences are if you don't ask them? And if you ask them, how will you know how to handle the information you get back?

Carrying out consultations using a shared decision-making approach can be challenging (Elwyn et al., 2017). To help clinicians develop skills in shared decision-making, the AHRQ has developed a number of tools to help with the process (AHRQ, 2014). They suggest a five-step process for structuring a shared decision-making consultation, known as SHARE:

Step 1: **S**eek your patient's participation.
Step 2: **H**elp your patient explore and compare treatment options.
Step 3: **A**ssess your patient's values and preferences.
Step 4: **R**each a decision with your patient.
Step 5: **E**valuate your patient's decision.

Another framework for shared decision-making, the three-talk model, was originally developed in 2012 and then revised in 2017 (Elwyn et al., 2012, 2017) (Fig. 9.6). This framework proposes a three-stage process or model (acknowledging that a consultation process may be iterative rather than linear) incorporating the following elements:

1. Team talk—working together to describe choices, offer support, and ask about patient goals.
2. Option talk—discussing alternatives, using risk communication principles.
3. Decision talk—identifying informed preferences and making preference-based decisions.

The authors emphasize the importance of active listening, ensuring that you are paying attention to what the patient is saying and responding appropriately, and thinking carefully about the different treatment options when facing a decision (deliberation) (Elwyn et al., 2017).

Although the two models have different numbers of stages, they both emphasize key elements of a shared decision-making consultation. This includes ensuring that you start the conversation by exploring what the patient wants to achieve (summarizing what his or her problem might

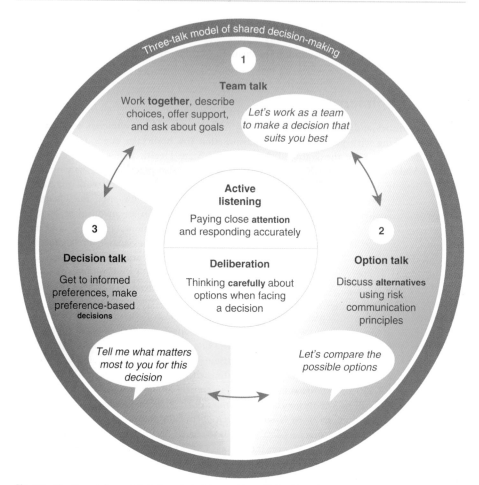

Fig. 9.6 The three-talk model of shared decision-making, 2017. (From Elwyn, G., Durand, M.A., Song, J., Aarts, J., Barr, P.J., Berger, Z., et al., 2017. A three-talk model for shared decision making: multistage consultation process. BMJ 359, j4891, with permission.)

be, asking the patient to participate in the decision-making process, and exploring the different treatment options available), explicitly discussing the benefits and harms of each available option (using risk communication principles such as those discussed later in this chapter), and exploring your patient's values and preferences associated with different treatment options, before reaching an agreed decision or decisions.

Both frameworks provide general guidance on sharing information and developing a shared understanding of the decision problem, which can help you involve patients in the decision process, as well as hopefully engage them with research evidence. To achieve this, you will also need to be able to fully explain the results of research studies to patients.

Explaining Evidence to Patients

If patients are to make informed decisions about their care, they will need to understand what the risks and benefits are of the different options available to them. Your role will be to take the evidence from different types of research studies and communicate it to patients either to help them evaluate their preferences for different options, or as a way of encouraging a more shared decision.

How we communicate information to patients can affect the decisions they make. Often when we are faced with healthcare decisions, we can look at potential outcomes in terms of likelihood of positive outcomes (e.g., survival) or negative outcomes (e.g., mortality). How we discuss these outcomes (known as "framing") can have a significant impact on an individual's choice. Gong et al. carried out a systematic review of studies examining how framing affected healthcare decision choices (Gong et al., 2013). They found that when potential outcomes were expressed positively (e.g., survival) people were more likely to choose more invasive treatments such as surgery. In studies that look at changes in health behavior (e.g., weight loss or smoking cessation), individuals were more likely to change their behavior in the desired direction when potential outcomes were expressed in terms of gains to health. Health professionals need to communicate the likelihood of different outcomes occurring to patients without unduly influencing their choices. To maintain an objective approach when communicating different options, information should be framed both positively and less positively.

How individuals understand risks and benefits differs, meaning that you may need to communicate the same information in different ways. Verbal descriptions, numerical presentations, and graphs and charts may all have a place in the communication of information to patients.

In general, it is probably better not to use verbal terms such as "rarely" or "sometimes" to explain the likelihood of outcomes occurring. This is because different individuals attach different meanings to the same verbal terms. For example seminal studies exploring doctors' and patients' interpretations of risk expressions found that doctors interpreted the verbal expression "extremely rare" to mean that an event occurred in a range between 0% of the time and 15% of the time and that there is a mismatch in understanding between professionals and patients (Shaw and Dear, 1990; Timmermans et al., 2004).

For this reason, it is generally better to try and communicate the potential risks and benefits associated with different treatment options using numerical or graphical means. Numerical presentation of results of research studies include absolute risk, relative risk, and number needed to treat. Absolute and relative risk can be communicated as percentages, probabilities, or natural frequencies. Based on a number of reviews examining the effect of different presentations of risk on an individual's understanding of risk (Akl et al., 2011; Fagerlin et al., 2011; Ahmed et al., 2012; Naik et al., 2012; Edwards et al., 2013), it has been suggested that when communicating risk you should:

- use natural frequencies (e.g., this outcome occurs in 2 in 100 people just like you) rather than percentages or probabilities (e.g., this outcome occurs in 2% or 0.02 people just like you)
- use absolute risk values (i.e., the observed or calculated risk or rate of an event occurring in a defined population) rather than relative risk values (which compare the risk or rate of an event in two different groups of people). For example, say: "the risk of a non-smoking woman developing breast cancer is 1 in 100" rather than: "there is a 50% increase in the risk of developing breast cancer if you smoke"
- give an idea of the baseline level of risk where appropriate (e.g., "the risk of you developing breast cancer over the next 10 years if you do not stop smoking is 2 in 100")
- use the same denominator across all the frequency information that you provide, so for example, if presenting data for two groups, use the denominator of 100 in both groups
- personalize the information so that it is based on the individual's own risk factors

Many individuals have problems understanding numeric information, so you may also need to consider providing information about risks and benefits graphically. The choice of graph you could use, and its applicability, depend on the type of information you are trying to convey (see Fig. 9.7 for examples). Stick-figures or faces (icon displays) are useful for giving individuals information about their risk of developing a condition over time and how

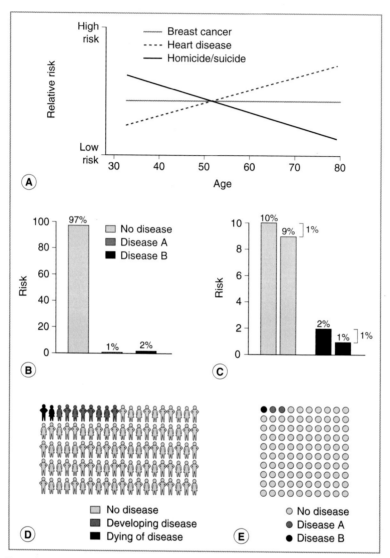

Fig. 9.7 Examples of graphical representations of risk. A: Line graph indicating relative risk of disease by age B: Bar graph of absolute risk C: Bar graph of relative risk D: Stick figures of risk of developing and dying of disease E: Icon display of risk of disease. (From Thompson, C., Dowding, D., 2009. Essential Decision Making and Clinical Judgement for Nurses. Edinburgh: Elsevier, 242–243, with permission.)

that risk may alter if they change their behavior (Fagerlin et al., 2011). The risk calculator QRISK provides a good example of this approach (www.qrisk.org; QRISK uses information about your current health status to provide you with a risk of developing heart disease or stroke over 10 years. This information is presented as a natural frequency, percentage and using an icon display. Other types of graphical display include bar graphs (for comparison of efficacy of treatments), line graphs (for displaying information on risks of an event over time), and pie charts (to show the proportion of individuals at risk of developing a condition) (Garcia-Retamero and Cokely, 2017). How information is presented to individuals needs to be tailored both to their preferences and their ability to understand the information you are

---

> **BOX 9.4 ■ Main Components of a Patient Decision Aid**
>
> ■ Explicitly state the decision that is being considered.
> ■ Provision of evidence-based information about health condition, the options, associated benefits, harms, probabilities, and scientific uncertainties.
> ■ Assistance to help patients to recognize the value-sensitive nature of the decision and to clarify, either implicitly or explicitly, the value they place on the benefits, harms, and scientific uncertainties. Strategies that may be included in the decision aid are: describing the options in enough detail that clients can imagine what it is like to experience the physical, emotional, and social effects; and guiding clients to consider which benefits and harms are most important to them.
>
> ---
>
> From Stacey, D., Légaré, F., Lewis, K., Barry, M.J., Bennett, C.L., Eden, K.B., et al., 2017. Decision aids for people facing health treatment or screening decisions. Cochrane Database Syst. Rev. (4), CD001431.

---

giving them. Note too, that the format that individuals may prefer may not necessarily be the format that enables them to fully understand the information they are being provided (Garcia-Retamero and Cokely, 2017).

Decision Aids and Decision Support

One of the main ways in which research evidence can be used effectively to assist with decision-making, both for clinicians and patients as a way of supporting through the process, is through the use of tools such as decision aids and decision support. It is important to distinguish between the two, as their focus and purpose differ. Decision support tools are normally developed for use by clinicians, whereas decision aids (Box 9.4) are normally designed to be used by patients (either with or without clinician input) to supplement the decision-making process. Both decision support tools and decision aids can be an effective way of helping to incorporate evidence from research into the decision process.

Clinical decision support (CDS) tools can be paper- or computer-based. They incorporate evidence from research to provide clinicians with guidance for a specific clinical decision. Jaspers et al. carried out a synthesis of systematic reviews clinical decision support systems, which identified 17 high-quality reviews that evaluated the effectiveness of such tools in practice (Jaspers et al., 2011). Overall, the reviews represented 229 individual studies. The types of decisions they support include diagnosis, public health interventions (e.g., vaccination), and medication decisions. Decision support has perhaps had its greatest impact in the area of medications guidance, in particular, in preventing drug interactions and overdose. The use of decision support tools in nursing is not common but is increasing. For example, CDS tools have been developed to assist with nursing assessment/diagnosis (e.g., cancer pain management, delirium identification), medication management, situational awareness (e.g. transplant management, sepsis alerting), guideline adherence, triage, and non–medication-based nursing interventions (Dunn Lopez et al., 2017).

The evidence base for decision support in nursing is not as robust as that in medicine. An integrative review of the evidence for the use of CDS in nursing in acute settings found that only 7 of the 22 studies included in the review reported process outcome changes, and 5 of the 22 reported patient outcomes (Dunn Lopez et al., 2017). These studies provide mixed results, with improvements in patient outcomes such as blood sugar and potassium regulation, and no change in outcomes for resource utilization.

In contrast, decision aids are resources specifically designed to help patients to make choices regarding the treatment options when there is no one obvious "best" option (Stacey et al., 2017). They can be used before, during, or after consultations with clinicians to help patients become actively involved in the decisions about their care. Decision aids can also be used as a way of facilitating shared decision-making (Stacey et al., 2017). A systematic review of the impact of decision aids on patient decision-making suggests that the aids can improve knowledge, reduce the amount of conflict patients feel about the decision process, and help individuals to reach a decision (Stacey et al., 2017). When decision aids incorporate specific information about the probabilities related to outcomes, they improve the accuracy of individuals' risk perceptions (Stacey et al., 2017). The use of decision aids may also affect the types of choices that patients make, such as reducing invasive surgery, reducing PSA screening, and increasing the likelihood of starting new medications for diabetes (Stacey et al., 2017).

Decision aids vary in the information they contain and their quality. In an attempt to help patients and healthcare professionals evaluate decision aids, the International Patient Decision Aid Standards (IPDAS) Collaboration has produced a list of standards http://ipdas.ohri.ca/; If you are interested in trying to locate a decision aid for a particular condition, there is an online inventory of patient decision aids at http://decisionaid.ohri.ca/AZinvent.php.

Summary

This chapter provides an overview of various ways in which research evidence from studies on populations can be integrated into decision-making for individual patients. It is important to highlight that the evidence from research is often only one of many factors that need to be taken into account when making healthcare decisions, and that issues such as patient preferences and ensuring that patients are included in the decision process are equally important issues to address wherever appropriate. You are encouraged to undertake more in-depth reading using the resources listed, and to practice using decision support tools. You can also consolidate your learning from this chapter by undertaking the online exercises.

References

Agency for Healthcare Research and Quality, 2014. The SHARE approach—essential steps of shared decisionmaking: quick reference guide. Available from: http://www.ahrq.gov/professionals /education/curriculum-tools/shareddecisionmaking/tools/tool-1/index.html (Accessed 9.4.18.).

Ahmed, H., Naik, G., Willoughby, H., Edwards, A.G., 2012. Communicating risk. BMJ 344, e3996.

Akl, E.A., Oxman, A.D., Herrin, J., Vist, G.E., Terrenato, I., Sperati, F., et al., 2011. Using alternative statistical formats for presenting risks and risk reductions. Cochrane Database Syst. Rev. 3, CD006776.

Benner, P., 1984. From Novice to Expert: Excellence and Power in Clinical Nursing Practice. Addison-Wesley, Reading, MA.

Benner, P., Tanner, C., 1987. How expert nurses use intuition. Am. J. Nurs. 87 (1), 23–31.

Daley, A., Stokes-Lampard, H., Thomas, A., MacArthur, C., 2014. Exercise for vasomotor menopausal symptoms. Cochrane Database Syst. Rev. 11, CD006108.

Dowding, D., Thompson, C., 2009. Evidence based decisions: the role of decision analysis. Essential decision making and judgement for nurses. Elsevier, Edinburgh, UK, p. 173–196.

Dunn Lopez, K., Gephart, S.M., Raszewski, R., Sousa, V., Shehorn, L.E., Abraham, J., 2017. Integrative review of clinical decision support for registered nurses in acute care settings. J. Am. Med. Inform. Assoc. 24 (2), 441–450.

Edwards, A.G.K., Naik, G., Ahmed, H., Elwyn, G.J., Pickles, T., Hood, K., et al., 2013. Personalised risk communication for informed decision making about taking screening tests. Cochrane Database Syst. Rev. (2), CD001865.

Elstein, A.S., Shulman, L.S., Sprafka, S.A., 1978. Medical Problem Solving: An Analysis of Clinical Reasoning. Harvard University Press, Cambridge, MA.

Elwyn, G., Durand, M.A., Song, J., Aarts, J., Barr, P.J., Berger, Z., et al., 2017. A three-talk model for shared decision making: multistage consultation process. BMJ 359, j4891.

Elwyn, G., Frosch, D., Thomson, R., Joseph-Williams, N., Lloyd, A., Kinnersley, P., et al., 2012. Shared decision making: a model for clinical practice. J. Gen. Intern. Med. 27 (10), 1361–1367.

Evans, J. St.B.T., 2011. Dual-process theories of reasoning: contemporary issues and developmental applications. Dev. Rev. 31 (2-3), 86–102.

Fagerlin, A., Zikmund-Fisher, B.J., Ubel, P.A., 2011. Helping patients decide: ten steps to better risk communication. J. Natl. Cancer Inst. 103 (19), 1436–1443.

Garcia-Retamero, R., Cokely, E.T., 2017. Designing visual aids that promote risk literacy: a systematic review of health research and evidence-based design heuristics. Hum. Factors 59 (4), 582–627.

Gigerenzer, G., Gaissmaier, W., 2011. Heuristic decision making. Ann. Rev. Psychol. 62, 451–482.

Gillespie, B.M., Chaboyer, W., St John, W., Morley, N., Nieuwenhoven, P., 2015. Health professionals' decision-making in wound management: a grounded theory. J. Adv. Nurs. 71 (6), 1238–1248.

Gong, J., Zhang, Y., Yang, Z., Huang, Y., Feng, J., Zhang, W., 2013. The framing effect in medical decision-making: a review of the literature. Psychol. Health Med. 18 (6), 645–653.

Hunink, M.G.M., Weinstein, M.C., Wittenberg, E., Drummond, M.F., Pliskin, J.S., Wong, J.B., et al., 2014. Decision Making in Health and Medicine: Integrating Evidence and Values. Cambridge University: Press Cambridge, MA.

Jaspers, M.W., Smeulers, M., Vermeulen, H., Peute, L.W., 2011. Effects of clinical decision-support systems on practitioner performance and patient outcomes: a synthesis of high-quality systematic review findings. J. Am. Med. Inform. Assoc. 18 (3), 327–334.

Jefford, E., Fahy, K., Sundin, D., 2011. Decision-making theories and their usefulness to the midwifery profession both in terms of midwifery practice and the education of midwives. Int. J. Nurs. Pract. 17 (3), 246–253.

Kahneman, D., 2013. Thinking, Fast and Slow. Farrar, Straus and Giroux, New York, NY.

Lamond, D., Crow, R., Chase, J., 1996. Judgements and processes in care decisions in acute medical and surgical wards. J. Eval. Clin. Pract. 2 (3), 211–216.

MacLennan, A.H., Broadbent, J.L., Lester, S., Moore, V., 2004. Oral oestrogen and combined oestrogen/progestogen therapy versus placebo for hot flushes. Cochrane Database Syst. Rev. (4), CD002978.

Marjoribanks, J., Farquhar, C., Roberts, H., Lethaby, A., Lee, J., 2017. Long-term hormone therapy for perimenopausal and postmenopausal women. Cochrane Database Syst. Rev. 1, CD004143.

Marwala, T., Hurwitz, E., 2017. Bounded Rationality. Artificial Intelligence and Economic Theory: Skynet in the Market. Springer, Cham, Switzerland.

Naik, G., Ahmed, H., Edwards, A.G., 2012. Communicating risk to patients and the public. Br. J. Gen. Pract. 62 (597), 213–216.

North American Association of Central Cancer Registries, 2018. NAACCR Fast Stats. 2010-2014 Cancer Incidence Data. Available from: https://faststats.naaccr.org/selections.php? (Accessed 19.3.18.).

O'Connor, A., Wells, G., Tugwell, P., et al., 1999. The effects of an "explicit" values clarification exercise in a woman's decision aid regarding postmenopausal hormone therapy. Health Expect 2 (1), 21–32.

Patterson, J., Skinner, J., Foureur, M., 2015. Midwives' decision making about transfers for "slow" labour in rural New Zealand. Midwifery 31 (6), 606–612.

Shafir, A., Rosenthal, J., 2012. Shared Decision-Making: Advancing Patient Centered Care through State and Federal Implementation. National Academy for State Health Policy, Portland, ME.

Shaw, N.J., Dear, P.R., 1990. How do parents of babies interpret qualitative expressions of probability? Arch. Dis. Child. 65 (5), 520.

Simmons, B., 2010. Clinical reasoning: concept analysis. J. Adv. Nurs. 66 (5), 1151–1158.

Siu, A.L., U.S. Preventive Services Task Force (USPSTF), 2016. Screening for breast cancer: U.S. Preventive Services task force recommendation statement. Ann. Intern. Med. 164 (4), 279–296.

Stacey, D., Légaré, F., Lewis, K., Barry, M.J., Bennett, C.L., Eden, K.B., et al., 2017. Decision aids for people facing health treatment or screening decisions. Cochrane Database Syst. Rev. (4), CD001431.

Thompson, C., Dowding, D., 2009. Essential Decision Making and Clinical Judgement for Nurses. Elsevier, Edinburgh.

Thompson, C., McCaughan, D., Cullum, N., Sheldon, T.A., Mulhall, A., Thompson, D.R., 2001. Research information in nurses' clinical decision-making: what is useful? J. Adv. Nurs. 36 (3), 376–388.

Thompson, C., Cullum, N., McCaughan, D., Sheldon, T., Raynor, P., 2004. Nurses, information use, and clinical decision making—the real world potential for evidence-based decisions in nursing. Evid. Based Nurs. 7 (3), 68–72.

Timmermans, D., Molewijk, B., Stiggelbout, A., Kievit, J., 2004. Different formats for communicating surgical risks to patients and the effect on choice of treatment. Patient Educ. Couns. 54 (3), 255–263.

Witteman, H.O., Gavaruzzi, T., Scherer, L.D., Pieterse, A.H., Fuhrel-Forbis, A., Chipenda Dansokho, S., et al., 2016. Effects of design features of explicit values clarification methods: a systematic review. Med. Decis. Making 36 (6), 760–776.

Yang, H., Thompson, C., Bland, M., 2012. The effect of clinical experience, judgment task difficulty and time pressure on nurses' confidence calibration in a high fidelity clinical simulation. BMC Med. Inform. Decis. Mak. 12, 113.

Yost, J., Ganann, R., Thompson, D., Aloweni, F., Newman, K., Hazzan, A., et al., 2015. The effectiveness of knowledge translation interventions for promoting evidence-informed decision-making among nurses in tertiary care: a systematic review and meta-analysis. Implement. Sci. 10, 98.

Yost, J., Thompson, D., Ganann, R., Aloweni, F., Newman, K., McKibbon, A., et al., 2014. Knowledge translation strategies for enhancing nurses' evidence-informed decision making: a scoping review. Worldviews Evid. Based Nurs. 11 (3), 156–167.

Further Reading/Internet Resources

Gigerenzer, G., 2002. Reckoning with Risk: Learning to Live with Uncertainty. Penguin Books, London.
> An easy-to-read introduction.
> An easy-to-read introduction into the fallibility of human reasoning and how to interpret research evidence.

Hunink, M.G.M., Weinstein, M.C., Wittenberg, E., Drummond, M.F., Pliskin, J.S., Wong, J.B., et al., 2014. Decision Making in Health and Medicine: Integrating Evidence and Values. Cambridge University Press, Cambridge, MA.
> A good overview.
> A good overview of the process of decision analysis.

Thompson, C., Dowding, D., 2009. Essential Decision Making and Clinical Judgement for Nurses. Elsevier, Edinburgh.
> More detailed discussion.
> More detailed discussion of the issues raised here, as well as an overview of decision making in nursing.

Online inventory of patient decision aids: http://decisionaid.ohri.ca/AZinvent.php

Online calculator for Bayes' theorem: http://araw.mede.uic.edu/cgi-bin/testcalc.pl

CHAPTER 10

How Can We Develop an Evidence-Based Culture?

Carl Thompson ■ Patricia Quinlan

KEY POINTS

- Evidence-based cultures promote decisions that appropriately weight research evidence, patient preference, available resources and clinical expertise at all levels of healthcare systems.
- Successful strategies for promoting evidence-based culture are likely to be multifaceted but targeted at specific cultural groups in organizations.
- The identification of groups for targeted and planned change interventions is best achieved through effective strategies.
- Theoretical models can help with planning and evaluating structured change strategies.
- Almost all professional behavioral interventions have *some* effect on practice – of interest is whether change happens by chance, or design.
- Audit and feedback approaches such as "benchmarking", although common, have a mixed and unpredictable impact on changing professional behavior and culture.

Introduction

Culture shapes the beliefs and behaviors of those delivering health care. If culture is ignored when implementing research evidence, strategies for change will almost certainly fail. But cultural change is unpredictable (Mannion and Smith, 2018). Real-world evidence-based change in organizations requires well-planned, targeted, informed strategies that incorporate what we know about both culture and the foreseeable effects of general and specific change interventions. Organizations such as the Department of Veterans Affairs (VA), Agency for Healthcare Research and Quality (AHRQ) in the US, and Health Services Delivery Research program within the National Institute for Health Research (NIHR HSDR) in the UK have funded research that has extended our empirical and theoretical knowledge considerably since previous editions of this book. This chapter aims to steer a course through some of these developments.

National Imperatives

Individual professional groups are striving to foster evidence-based decision-making as part of their professional cultures and norms. Registered nurses have a professional duty to practice effectively based on the best available evidence (Nursing and Midwifery Council, 2018; Canadian Nurses Association, 2017; Nursing and Midwifery Board of Australia, 2016; Nursing Council of New Zealand, 2012). In the US, the American Nurses Association (ANA) views evidence-based care as the "cornerstone" of nursing practice (American Nurses Association, 2015). Knowledge transfer includes meticulous review of scientific evidence combined with nurse experience and patient preferences to provide exemplary patient care services.

Nurses work within wider, national policy systems. Greater use of scientific knowledge in improving the quality of health services is a policy objective for almost all developed countries. The following are examples from the US to illustrate this point:

- The AHRQ, a federal sub-agency of the U.S. Department of Health and Human Services, fosters evidence-based health care through a myriad of evaluative initiatives (www.ahrq.gov). One example is the use of information technology intended to improve health care and reduce inequalities.
- The Joint Commission—as an agent of the Center for Medicare and Medicaid Services (www.jointcommission.org)—promotes the use of scientific evidence by requiring organizations to report "core" performance measures. These process measures reflect adherence to practices known to be associated with good patient outcomes. Performance on these metrics tied to financial reimbursement further incentivizes a cultural shift to the application of best practice (Chassin et al., 2010; Chassin and Loeb, 2013). The Joint Commission further fosters adoption of EBP through its Top Performer on Key Quality Measures program. This program recognizes accredited hospitals achieving excellence on performance measures specific to evidence-based interventions.
- The Institute of Medicine (IOM) Roundtable on Evidence-Based Medicine is a professional structure with an ambition that 90% of clinical decisions will be supported by accurate, timely, and up-to-date clinical information by 2020 (Institute of Medicine, 2010). Beginning with, "To Err is Human: Building a Safer Health Care System" (Institute of Medicine, 2000) and then with the nursing focused, "Keeping Patients Safe: Transforming the Work Environment of Nurses"(Page, 2004), the IOM has led efforts for a cultural shift in patient and clinician expectations of safety. That shift depends in part on creating tools such as protocols for care that are evidence based, and an honest look at safety culture within an organization. AHRQ's own self-assessment instruments can be used to evaluate staff perceptions of the safety climate where they work (https://www.ahrq.gov/sops/surveys/index.html. Permission required for use outside of US).

The Institute for Health Improvement uses an approach termed "science of improvement" to shape cultures and optimize health care delivery. Interventions based on high-quality randomized evidence are incorporated into care process "bundles" that seek to improve clinical outcomes. Bundles are applied repeatedly and carefully so that all component parts are used and outcomes evaluated; the result is habitual and reliable deployment of the beneficial practice (Resar et al., 2005).

Similarly in the UK, the National Health Service (NHS) has a legal obligation to promote research and the use of research evidence in its service commissioning, provision, and delivery (NHS England, 2017). In brief, NHS Trust boards have a formal duty to ensure that quality is improved, and bodies such as the National Institute for Health and Care Excellence (NICE), and the Care Quality Commission, exist to monitor and support this duty.

What Does an Evidence-Based Culture Look Like?

The key components of an evidence-based culture are well established and have not changed substantively since the mid-1990s:

> *"built-in … capability to generate, and the flexibility to incorporate, evidence and individuals and teams who can find, appraise and use research evidence."*

(MUIR GRAY, 1997)

BOX 10.1 ▣ Ten Key Features of Organizational Culture

Attitudes to innovation and risk taking

The degree to which the organization encourages and rewards new ways of doing things or, conversely, values tradition

Degree of central direction

The extent of central setting of objectives and performance versus devolved decision-making

Patterns of communication

The degree to which instruction and reporting are channeled via formal hierarchies rather than informal networks

Outcome or process orientation

Whether the organization values (focuses on) outcomes and results as opposed to tasks

Internal or external focus

Whether the organization looks inward and restricts itself to organizational issues as opposed to looking at the needs of customers

Uniformity or diversity

The organizational propensity toward consistency or diversity

People orientation

Valuation of the human resources available to an organization

Team orientation

Does the organization reward individualism or is it geared more toward teamwork?

Aggressiveness/competitiveness

The extent to which the organization seeks to dominate or cooperate with external competitors or players

Attitudes to change

The extent to which the organization demonstrates a predilection for stability in preference to dynamic change

---

Modified from Davies, H.T., Nutley, S.M., Mannion, R., 2000. Organisational culture and quality of health care. Qual. Health Care 9 (2), 111–119.

Davies et al. suggest 10 targets for organizational culture change to promote aims that might include evidence-based decisions (Davies et al., 2000) (Box 10.1).

To realize this cultural change capability, organizations depend on interdependent systems that promote evidence-based decisions accompanied by supportive structures and processes that are effective and efficient. Before trying to change the culture of an organization or unit, some key uncertainties must be tackled: most importantly, understanding and establishing why change is required and who and what can change.

Diagnosing the Challenges to Changing Practice—Understanding Complexity

Changing cultures is complex (Braithwaite et al., 2017), and understanding this complexity takes time. Various frameworks have been put forward to ease the task faced by the clinician or manager in planning change in complex environments. Examples include the 7s model, soft systems methodology, content context and process modeling, and the "5 Whys" (Iles and Sutherland, 2001). The "5 Whys" approach (with its roots in Aristotelian philosophy) is particularly useful for

> **BOX 10.2 ■ The "5 Whys" Approach to Understanding Complexity**
>
> **Problem** Nurses are routinely ordering (unnecessary) urine tests on children who do not require them.
>
> **Why does this happen?** It is seen as a necessary routine part of admission screening.
>
> **Why?** Nurses do not understand the clinical value of looking at signs and symptoms and prevalence alongside the "dipstick" urinalysis test they undertake.
>
> **Why?** Nurses do not know about the positive predictive value of a test such as urinalysis.
>
> **Why?** Nurses do not know what "positive predictive value" means and how to estimate it "on the fly" in routine practice.
>
> **Why?** Because they have not been introduced to the concept in practice and had its application reinforced.

making sense of problems (see Box 10.2); in essence it simply involves asking the question "why?" and then continuing to ask why in response to the answers generated. It is low-tech but effective, and it has a 2500 year old provenance!

Any approach to simplifying complexity should:

- identify all the groups involved in, affected by, or influencing the proposed change(s) in practice
- assess characteristics of the proposed change that might influence its adoption
- assess the preparedness of people to change, and other potentially relevant internal factors within the target group
- identify potential external barriers to change
- identify likely enabling factors, including resources and skills (NHS CRD 1999)

Approaches require data as the means of providing answers to questions generated. One theory and organizing framework, with an expanding library of applications, is Normalization Process Theory (NPT) (May et al., 2007, 2009). NPT explains and predicts how new things (technologies, innovations) become part of routine work. It seeks answers to four key questions to understand a problem and help generate planned solutions:

- What is the work involved?
- Who gets to do the work?
- How does the work get done?
- How is the work understood?

NPT has a toolkit to help healthcare professionals think about these questions and gather the right data (May et al., 2015).

Surveys are useful, but what people say they do (or will do) and how they behave (or will behave) are often at odds. Techniques that generate more observational, socially located data can be useful, such as:

- ward meetings or clinical supervision sessions adapted so that potential problems can be identified, recorded, and fed into the strategic planning process.
- focus groups of professionals, managers, and, where appropriate, patients or their representatives, to identify barriers and drivers to cultural change. Cameron and Wren used this approach (Cameron and Wren, 1999) by forming "buzz" groups of 6 to 8 people who used "reflection-on-action" (Schön, 1994) to identify their values. These were typed and distributed to the group who then worked toward a collective understanding of the values identified.

Newhouse reviewed instruments for measuring organizational capacity for EBP (Newhouse, 2010). Studies included looked at vision, leadership, and learning culture as well as stages of knowledge transfer such as acquisition of new knowledge, knowledge sharing, and use.

Three instruments were highlighted as useful, internally consistent, and valid: (i) Context Assessment (McCormack et al., 2009), (ii) Alberta Context Tool (Estabrooks et al., 2009), and (iii) Organizational Readiness to Change Assessment (Helfrich et al., 2009).

How Can Evidence-Based Innovation and Culture Be Encouraged?

We have known for some time that no "magic bullets" exist for planned deliberate change based around using research evidence (Oxman et al., 1995). Although much is known about the ingredients that can be used in a change strategy (e.g., see the systematic reviews of the Cochrane Collaboration's Effective Practice and Organisation of Care [EPOC] group http://epoc.cochrane.org/), optimal combinations remain stubbornly elusive.

Three major dimensions must be addressed by anyone considering cultural change, as evidenced by changes in behavior:

- The innovation itself
- The individuals and groups involved
- The system in which the innovation must operate

None of these three elements operates in isolation, so a fourth dimension can be added to this list:

- The linkages (between the innovation, the system, and the individuals involved).

THE INNOVATION

Those characteristics of the innovation associated with positive uptake in organizations are highlighted in Box 10.3.

THE INDIVIDUAL

Individuals work creatively with their organizations, and the individual differences that mark out team members also extend to the ways in which they interact with innovations. To maximize the chances of change adoption by a team and its members, it is important to understand those characteristics of individuals, teams, and the unit involved (Box 10.4).

THE ORGANIZATION AS A KNOWLEDGE-DRIVEN SYSTEM

Using management to develop an organization's structural and cultural components is a necessary step in encouraging assimilation of evidence-based innovations. The structural components of an organization and their relationship to innovativeness (a key component of an evidence-based culture) are summarized in Table 10.1.

As Table 10.1 shows, some elements of culture can be manipulated in an organization's drive to innovate. Although not all parts of an organizational system can be directly controlled by clinicians or individual managers, they are still important elements of context to be borne in mind when developing change strategies.

Another important antecedent for developing an evidence-based culture at the level of systems is the organization's capacity for absorbing new knowledge. Knowledge in service organizations underpins the degree to which an organization can codify what it does, capture new information, and design it into work practices and the decision-making machinery. This is an important determinant of the service that the public eventually receives (Ashburner, 2001; Kash et al., 2013).

BOX 10.3 ▪ Attributes of an Innovation Associated with Adoption

Standard or universal attributes

Relative advantage

The degree to which there is a clear and unambiguous effectiveness or cost-effectiveness advantage beyond "where we are now," remembering that the concept or idea of "advantage" is sometimes socially constructed via negotiation between stakeholders (for example, one person's timesaving computerized shortcut may be another's day away from practice learning to use unfamiliar and confusing software).

Compatibility

Fit with the values and norms of the workplace

Complexity

Simple (or the ability to break down the innovation into a simple form) equates with higher chances

Trialability

Can the innovation be tried out and experimented within the workplace?

Observability

Observable benefits increase adoption

Reinvention

The ability to shape an innovation to suit one's own needs equates to a higher chance of adoption

Operational or context-specific attributes

Innovation

Has to be seen as relevant for the adopter's work tasks

Performance improving

An innovation should be seen to improve performance in a given task

Perceived feasibility

In a given context

Divisibility

The ability to break it down into manageable components

Codified and transferable knowledge

The degree to which the knowledge needed to actually make use of the innovation can be separated from one context and transferred to another

---

Data become information and information becomes knowledge in line with contextual circumstances. Access to a store of good-quality information, relevant for the specific work setting, allows the scarce time for consulting "formal" (i.e., written) sources of information to be maximized. The necessary IT and digital resources to manage information are now commonplace. Elsewhere this book discusses searching for and appraisal of material. In particular, Chapter 3 highlights key resources that bring together professional judgment and research evidence in an accessible medium as well as ways that this provision of information might be facilitated through organizational structures. The cognitive benefits from consulting good-quality evidence can reinforce information-seeking behavior, helping to promote a learning culture.

The knowledge that shapes healthcare actions is socially constructed. For example, a particular drug may objectively be "effective," but, the decision on whether to administer the drug can change according to circumstance. Patient values, available resources, and the expertise of the health care professional involved all vary from context to context and can be negotiated by the parties involved. Once the contested nature of the knowledge required for managing decisions

---

BOX 10.4 ■ Adopting Change: Considerations at the Level of the Individual

Psychological precursors

Cognitive and social psychology literature suggests that the degree to which someone is tolerant of ambiguity, their intellect, and their general values toward change will influence their propensity for trying new ideas. If the individual has identified a need and the innovation meets that need, then change is more likely.

Meaning

The meaning that an innovation may have for an adopter needs to be established. If this meaning fits the meaning associated with management and other stakeholding groups, then adopting an innovation is more likely.

Adoption decision nature

Is the decision to opt into the innovation contingent (i.e., does it depend on someone else in the organization?) or authoritative (a compulsory activity). Although authoritative decisions may appear to increase the chances of initial adoption, they also reduce the chances of long-term adoption.

Adoption decision stage concerns

It is important to remember that adoption is a process rather than a single event. Different concerns arise at different points in this process:

- Before adoption—individuals need to be aware of the pending change and be given enough information to decide how it will affect them.
- During the early stages—training and support to a level that will enable individuals to shape the change to their own working practices must be provided.
- Once the change is established—feedback of the consequences enables individuals to continue to refine the innovation for their own environments.

TABLE 10.1 ■ The Relationship Between Characteristics of Organizations and Innovativeness of Organizations

Characteristics	Direction of Relationship with Innovativeness (Positive or Negative)
Administrative costs	+
Autonomy in decision-making	−
Degrees of professionalism and specialization	+
Extent of workers' participation in professional activity outside the organization	+
Degree of rule-following and procedures	No significant relationship
Number of different work units	+
Communication between units	+
Managerial attitude to change	+
Managers' experience	No significant relationship
Degree of professional knowledge in the organization	+
Resources in an organization that "go beyond the minimum" required to do the job	+
Number of specialties	+
Amount of technical resources	+
Number of (hierarchical) levels in the organization	No significant relationship

in health care is acknowledged, the importance of the science of communication, knowledge management, and transfer becomes apparent. As Greenhalgh et al. put it:

> *"...before it [knowledge] can contribute to organisational change initiatives, knowledge must be enacted and made social, entering into the stock of knowledge constructed and shared by other individuals. Knowledge depends for its circulation on interpersonal networks and will spread only when these social factors and barriers are overcome."*

GREENHALGH ET AL., 2005

Introducing new knowledge into an environment that is not receptive to change is likely to lead to failure. Trust developed by clearly defined norms and values drives individual and collective behavior (Kimber et al., 2012). Institutional trust encourages collaboration as employees know what is expected of them (Zhang et al., 2008). Though participants may have disparate views, trust enables staff to unite around decisions that are patient-centered and evidence-based.

Greenhalgh et al. suggest a number of indicators of receptive environments: (i) strong leadership skills; (ii) clear strategic vision accompanied by managerial relations that help support that vision; (iii) key staff with a sense of shared vision; (iv) a risk-taking environment where trialing ideas is supported; and (v) good systems of data capture (Greenhalgh et al., 2005). This last point is an essential component as data forms the basis of information, which through the addition of context, then becomes knowledge.

Organizations that promote change are flexible and supportive, creating an environment of inquiry, involvement, and accountability (Kavanagh and Ashkanasy, 2006). For example, in a study exploring implementation of evidence-based practice through interviews with staff at a healthcare provider site (Kimber et al., 2012), participants discussed the importance of effective leadership during the implementation processes to steer the transformation and inspire others to complete tasks and focus on deliverables. They emphasized the importance of both front-line and management staff in the change process being inclusive of different points of view, as well as having an appreciation of work roles and responsibilities.

Organizations set the tone for knowledge creation and use. For the right tone, they need the capacity to absorb knowledge and an incentive to use it (Denis and Lehoux, 2013). Markers of such capacity include:

- a climate of autonomy where decisions about workflow are developed across all employment levels
- expectations of independent problem solving at the point-of-care, fostering creative solutions and search for knowledge to assist this process
- the ability to self-govern autonomously, in order to be sufficiently nimble to facilitate the access and application of evidence
- collective resolution by work communities at the local level; this requires a culture of collaboration and flexibility to adapt evidence to organizational and patient benefit
- the ability to balance principles of standardization as well as creativity where participants manipulate their workflow, maintaining core researched evidence, without overreduction (Denis and Lehoux, 2013).

For many clinicians, the "linkages" that bring these elements together are the strategies and specific approaches adopted to create cultural and behavioral change.

How Can Change Happen?

DEVELOPING AN EVIDENCE-BASED CHANGE TOOLKIT

Up to this point, the chapter has focused on important components in a framework for considering complexity and innovation in healthcare settings. Thinking about these components is a necessary stage for shaping cultural change and forms a contextual backdrop for planned action.

All of these elements can be molded to some degree, but it is specific change interventions that provide the most commonly encountered approach to the behaviors, values, and goals that make up culture.

There is a surprising amount of research summarizing what we know about interventions for changing behavior and translating research knowledge into research-informed health care decisions. For a sense of the volume of high-quality primary and secondary evidence available, see http://epoc.cochrane.org/.

WHAT WORKS, WHAT DOESN'T, AND WHY?

The Cochrane Collaboration's EPOC group has produced a typology of approaches commonly used in behavior change strategies (Table 10.2). We will employ this to frame our discussion of what works.

Systematic reviews and "reviews of reviews" reveal that the effects of the various behavior change strategies are rather modest and sobering. The likely gains in performance may be far lower and more variable than is often assumed by those developing interventions. Moreover, simply combining interventions in the hope that "more will be better" does not default to greater effectiveness.

Johnson and May have substantially advanced our knowledge, not just of which interventions work but *why*. They examined previously published systematic reviews, and used Normalization Process Theory, introduced earlier in this chapter, to categorize approaches to changing behavior

TABLE 10.2 ■ **A Typology of Professional Behavior Change Interventions for Professionals**

Intervention Approach	Description
Patient-mediated interventions	Information collected from patients (such as PROMs) and given to the clinician to alter his or her practice
Audit and feedback	A summary of clinical performance over time derived from notes, observation, or routine data.
Educational outreach	Using a trained person to meet with clinicians to provide information (sometimes feedback)
Reminders	Information designed to prompt recall or specific behavior (including computerized clinical decision support)
Educational meetings	Participating in conferences, lectures, seminars, and workshops
Education material distribution	Distributing (in person or by mail or other means) published or printed evidence such as protocols and clinical guidelines
Local consensus processes	Getting clinicians/teams to agree that a problem is important and the approach to resolving it is appropriate
Local opinion leaders	Using people nominated by their peers as "influential" to shape opinion
Marketing	Using interviews, focus groups, or surveys of professionals to identify barriers to change and using results to design interventions to overcome them
Mass media	Using communication such as television or radio or leaflets, sometimes alongside other interventions, and often targeting a population of staff (e.g., all nurses in a hospital)

Modified from Cochrane Collaboration's Effective Practice and Organisation of Care (EPOC) group. EPOC Taxonomy. Available from: http://epoc.cochrane.org/epoc-taxonomy.

in healthcare professionals according to the possible mechanisms for effectiveness (Johnson and May, 2015). Of note, they indicated that multi-faceted interventions were, on balance, no more likely to be effective on performance or patient outcomes than single interventions, and that interventions were variably effective and differed, thus making the choice of interventions important. In the following sections, we use their analysis to examine the interventions often used by nurses and other health care staff to promote evidence-based culture and practice. We have attempted to present the interventions in order, from most to least (relatively) effective intervention. However, there is no clear-cut order; findings from the systematic reviews reported in the Johnson and May paper varied considerably for some interventions.

Patient-Mediated Interventions

With this approach, information is collected from patients and given to clinicians to try and alter practice. Findings suggest a positive effect on professional performance (shown in three of four reviews; the fourth, much earlier review emphasized uncertainty) and possibly on patient outcomes (investigated in two reviews; one showed effectiveness, and the other was unclear) when used as part of a multifaceted approach.

Patient-mediated interventions seem to trigger action by generating collective action among team members and reflexive monitoring in those exposed to the intervention.

Audit and Feedback

This approach, which relies on professionals collecting, measuring against standards, analyzing, and interpreting data, has positive effects on both professional practice and clinical outcomes when used as a standalone intervention (investigated in one review). When used as part of a multifaceted intervention, it appears to have positive effects on professional practice (12 out of 15 reviews showed positive effects, with the remaining reviews showing unclear effects), however the picture is mixed for patient outcomes (of six reviews, two were positive and three were equivocal, however one provided evidence of ineffectiveness).

When effective, audit and feedback fostered a coherent solution to the work and enabled cognitive participation, collective action, and reflexive monitoring on the part of professionals.

Educational Outreach

This popular approach, which entails disseminating research findings through the use of trained people meeting with clinicians, was deemed moderately effective. As a single intervention, it has positive effects on professional practice (in the two reviews that investigated this) and possibly on clinical outcomes (one review was positive, and the other revealed an unclear effect). However, as part of a multifaceted strategy, the effects are mixed, both for professional practice outcomes (of 12 reviews, eight were positive, one showed evidence of ineffectiveness, and three showed unclear effects) and for clinical outcomes (of seven reviews, one was positive, two provided evidence of ineffectiveness, and four were unclear).

When effective, educational outreach initiated cognitive participation, fostered the integration of context into planned collective action, and had a strong appraisal (individual and group levels) that encouraged reflexive monitoring among professionals.

Reminders

Reminders, when used alone, have mixed effects on professional practice (of 18 reviews, 12 were positive, four provided evidence of ineffectiveness, and two were equivocal) and patient outcomes (of eleven reviews, four were positive, two showed evidence of ineffectiveness, and five were unclear). There is a very similar mixed picture for reminders when used as part of a multifaceted approach with regard to their impact on professional performance (investigated in 15 reviews) and patient outcomes (investigated in seven reviews).

Where reminders successfully modified behavior, it was arguably down to their effects on fostering collective action (being workable and adapting to context) and the ways in which they encourage reflexivity in practitioners.

Educational Meetings

Participating in conferences, workshops, and seminars has been a mainstay of Continuing Professional Development (CPD) for professionals. However, it has been known for many years that CPD is only variably effective and that the predictors of success are unclear (Forsetlund et al., 2009). Johnson and May's analysis suggests that this variable success might be attributable to a limited range of NPT constructs addressed by educational meetings (Johnson and May, 2015). Educational meetings used in combination with other interventions appear to have a positive effect on professional performance (of 16 reviews, 11 were positive and five were equivocal). However their impact on professional practice and clinical outcomes, when used as a standalone intervention, is mixed (of four reviews investigating professional practice, three were positive, one showed evidence on ineffectiveness, and one was equivocal; of eight reviews investigating clinical outcomes, two were positive, one provided evidence of ineffectiveness, and five had mixed results).

Educational meetings might get professionals out of the clinical environment for a few hours but are perhaps only moderately impactful as a means of changing culture.

Distributing Educational Materials

Some readers may think that the answer to (expensive) educational meetings may lie in the (cheaper) distribution of educational materials as a means of catalyzing change. Johnson and May's analysis suggests not (Johnson and May, 2015). Distribution of educational materials as a solo intervention has variable impact on both professional performance (three reviews were positive, one showed evidence of ineffectiveness, and one was uncertain) and patient outcomes (similar mixed results were seen across five reviews). Similarly, when considered as part of a multi-faceted approach, impact on professional practice is mixed positive (11 reviews were positive, one showed evidence of ineffectiveness, and three were unclear), however impact on clinical outcomes is, if anything, more uncertain (five reviews were positive, two showed evidence of ineffectiveness, and four were unclear).

Although this approach may be easier than other approaches to internalize (fostering coherence) and to integrate into work settings, its overall effectiveness is decidedly uncertain.

Guidelines and Integrated Care Pathways

Evidence-based guidelines, discussed in Chapter 8, are particularly useful to guide organizational policy and procedure changes. They target behavioral and cultural change. Johnson and May suggest that multifaceted approaches to implementing guidelines may be the best approach, and that "diagnosing" the barriers to change may be time well spent and enhance the chances of success considerably (93.8% of interventions vs. 47.1%, $p = 0.04$) (Johnson and May, 2015; Chaillet et al., 2006).

Strategies such as integrated care pathways (ICPs) combine local systems and processes with guideline information, sometimes with reminders built into documentation and monitoring technologies. Often these form part of a larger-scale clinical audit. The label "integrated care pathways" contains a heterogeneous combination of interventions; something not lost on those who have sought to systematically review the evidence for their use (Allen et al., 2009). Some general conclusions can be offered based on a narrative overview of the studies (Allen et al., 2009). First, in relation to "what works and when," ICPs can:

- support proactive management and ensure clinical interventions and/or assessments are relevant and timely (for relatively predictable trajectories of care)

- promote adherence to guidelines or treatment protocols and reduce unwarranted variations in practice
- help improve documentation of treatment goals and communication between patients, carers, and health professionals
- improve physician agreement about treatment options
- support decision-making where they contain decision aids
- change professional behaviors in the desired direction, where there is scope for improvement or where roles are new

Given the opportunity costs involved in their construction and implementation, it is helpful that Allen et al. also highlight the potential downsides of ICPs:

- Service quality and efficiency gains in patient trajectories are not a given in services that are already using best evidence and where multidisciplinary working is well-established.
- Benefits are not equally spread between patient sub-groups (e.g., young vs. old).
- Cost-effectiveness is not guaranteed, perhaps because supporting mechanisms to underpin their implementation are needed. The costs of such mechanisms are often ignored and, when accounted for, can alter the cost-effectiveness of strategies (Thompson et al., 2016). This is particularly the case when ICP use requires a significant change in organizational culture.
- ICP documentation can produce unintended consequences and new kinds of error.

At the organizational level, pathways templated through an electronic medical record (EMR) are designed to inform clinical decision-making at both the organizational and point-of-care levels. Pathways built into the EMR configured by organizational teams include both informatics and clinical stakeholders to organize information and data screens in a manner most helpful to the practitioner. Screens display information needed for making collaborative care decisions. Decision-making support integrated into electronic databases linked to research evidence allows carers to ask clinical questions while navigating the electronic record during patient care or interdisciplinary rounds. The building of order sets and pathways encourages use of evidence to establish protocols collectively approved across services. The use of evidence neutralizes personal self-interest and shifts focus to what is best for patient care. Technological devices make searching for knowledge more accessible and likely utilized. Organizations vested in technology create a climate that fosters evidence access by clinicians who use smart phones and clinical apps to guide decision-making.

Fellowships

Although educational approaches for specific behaviors may have limited appeal, knowledge transfer practiced in a simulated situation or applied directly to the work environment may be more effective for learning, especially when accompanied by mentorship. The Texas Christian Center for Evidence Based Practice and Research, a collaborative center of the Joanna Briggs Institute, created an evidence-based practice fellowship program in 2011 across 21 participant organizations (Weeks et al., 2011). Designed by direct care and nurse researchers, the program consists of six sessions delivered over a 9-month period. Content includes both evidence-based fundamentals as well as guidance with project development, evaluation, and dissemination. Participating institutions invest resources such as paid time for fellows and mentors to complete the projects.

One evaluation of a point-of-care training program found significant changes in average knowledge and evidence-based practice ability after implementation of a curriculum focusing on knowledge translation (Black et al., 2015). Qualitative findings noted participants reported greater awareness of the link between practice and research with mentors seen as particularly invaluable.

Communication Strategies

Communicating evidence means replacing outdated information and knowledge with new current information and creating new knowledge. Clear, targeted, and explanatory communication helps convey why a change in practice is important and encourages adoption. Feedback on what is expected of practice helps validate understanding and normalizes change. Central digital systems of communication can help improve communication of, and access to, practice change information (Eppler and Mengis, 2009). Formal shared governance in the form of nurse-led evidence-based practice councils can help foster effective communication. In their study of six such councils, Brody et al. found that participants reported better communication of key practice information including why changes were important to patient care (Brody et al., 2012). Peer-generated communication via the council was also considered more valuable than communication by clinical educators.

Quality Improvement

Achieving change using quality frameworks is similar to the paradigms that guide evidence-based practice. One example of a framework that has proven useful in a range of quality and safety improvement contexts is Plan-Do-Study-Act (Lawton and Armitage, 2012) but others, each with varying levels of usefulness and evidence to support their use, include Six Sigma, Lean, Root Cause Analysis, and Failure Mode Analysis (Seidl and Newhouse, 2012). Quality improvement–rich organizations are familiar with introducing change and measuring the effect. The principle objective goal of quality improvement is to influence a process toward a desired impact, whereas a primary motivator of EBP is to transfer new knowledge and best practice (Sales, 2013). The strongest criticism of quality improvement is that data may not be representative of the issue under consideration. Problems that trigger the quality intervention tend to be local and need immediate action, and therefore the results of the initiative are not generalizable (Sales et al., 1995; Sales, 2013). Regardless, a culture that is knowledgeable and receptive about quality improvement is likely to absorb the deeper analytical approach associated with EBP.

One valuable resource for clinicians considering quality improvement in the US is the National Database of Nursing Quality Indicators (NDNQI). NDNQI is a nursing quality measurement program that enables hospitals to compare their performance on nursing-sensitive indicators with other national, regional, and state facilities. Organizations rely on NDNQI reporting to satisfy Magnet Recognition Program (discussed later) requirements. In addition to nursing-sensitive quality measures, NDNQI offers an annual satisfaction survey in which organizations can benchmark staff perceptions about their work environment. Participation in a benchmarking program serves to establish a culture of accountability, which is necessary to motivate use of evidence or systematic change.

Other Interventions in the EPOC Taxonomy

There are other interventions shown in Table 10.2 that clinicians could consider as part of a planned approach (e.g., marketing, opinion leaders), but their relative lack of effect or obvious advantages make detailed presentation of why they might work somewhat superfluous.

Real-Life Examples of Changing Practice and Culture

CASE 1: MAGNET DESIGNATION

The Magnet Program for Nursing Excellence recognizes organizations that can demonstrate that they strive for excellence (Graystone, 2017). Organizations must demonstrate how they apply and evaluate successful change within four evidence-based theoretical constructs in the

Magnet model: (i) transformational leadership, (ii) staff development, (iii) clinical practice, and (iv) generation and transfer of new knowledge and innovation. Data must show the effect of changes implemented and the embedding of best practice in 73 of the 153 sources of evidence that make up Magnet performance expectations. For example, organizations must demonstrate efforts toward a Bachelor of Science in Nursing as a minimum education standard, specialty certification, and visible strategies for ongoing improvement. The Magnet criterion of "New Knowledge and Innovation" specifically requires detailed examples of knowledge transfer and nursing research.

Magnet designation has cultural benefits. In a study carried out in Magnet and non-Magnet hospitals in New Jersey that compared RNs' skills in obtaining evidence ($N = 2911$, 32 hospitals), Magnet RNs reported significantly more: use of computers; information seeking from sources such as librarians and conferences; conducting evidence searches in CINAHL and MEDLINE; and greater identification, utilization, and participation in research. They were also more likely to rate their research-related resources as adequate or more than adequate (Cadmus et al., 2008). More recent surveys of 160 Magnet and non-Magnet facilities in the US found that Magnet organizations had nurses with more doctoral degrees and academic appointments; produced more research; provided more research mentors, practical research experience, and fellowship opportunities; and had a research governance structure specific to nursing research (McLaughlin et al., 2013).

The ANCC Magnet Program expects designated organizations to validate a culture that promotes research and evidence-based practice. These expectations increase with each revision of the application manual. Requirements include documented evidence of two nursing research studies, one completed and one in progress at the time of document submission. Conduct of research must include internal and external dissemination of study findings by clinical nurses. Four examples of evidence-based practice initiatives are required. Examples must detail search for evidence and the process of knowledge transfer. The use of evidence derived from multiple sources to inform organizational policy also is an obligatory exercise.

CASE 2: NATIONAL STANDARDS OR BENCHMARKS

In the course of teaching nurses about evidence-based health care, the comment is often made that evidence-based health care is only for the "technical" aspects of nursing or those roles that are seen as "cutting edge" in nursing and health care (such as the discipline of advanced practitioners). However, policy makers and the professions are using national standards or benchmarks alongside audit, education, and practice development to apply evidence-based principles to the essential aspects of patient care in areas such as maintaining privacy and dignity, communication, continence, and skin care. In the UK, the policy initiative, called the "essence of care" (Department of Health and Social Care, 2010), focuses on a series of standards (benchmarks) that are derived from research evidence and adjusted in response to structured consultation with patients, carers, and other stakeholders.

The benchmarks are designed to be tailored to local service delivery contexts via the PDSA framework (Plan, Do, Study, and Act), a technique for testing "change ideas." Review of the benchmarking data has exposed variations between services with respect to their location in the cycle of PDSA and resulted in systems that are planned, implemented, and evaluated with local context in mind.

The standards themselves are evidence based, represent policy concerns, and incorporate the values of users and the input of expert clinicians. The nature of the implementation process allows for trialing of the change ideas associated with progress toward the standards. The linkage to local and national audit processes allows for demonstration of progress (or lack of progress), a powerful driver in an era of competition among providers for patients and interprovider comparisons of performance. The standards have high degrees of work relevance and are designed to produce improved and visible task performance. Through the link with audit activity, there is the potential for feedback of task performance, and the standards provide frameworks for action that offer a degree of guidance for specific tasks associated with nursing roles.

Changes in the "culture" of the national workforce are much harder to demonstrate than changes in the activities of individuals or teams charged with implementing policy. Many of the UK reports on progress toward meeting these standards detail the "activity" that surrounds the implementation, for example, the establishment of a forum, the appointment of "champions," and the drafting of best practice. What is less common is the reporting of changes in patient outcome and workforce culture arising from the kind of multifaceted and targeted interventions that develop locally in response to national initiatives such as this.

CASE 3: USING THEORY EFFECTIVELY TO IMPROVE SAFETY AND SAFETY CULTURE

A team of academics (Taylor et al. 2013, 2014) worked with front-line improvement teams in three hospitals to implement national guidelines on nasogastric (NG) tube placement. The guideline recommends that the first-line method for confirming NG tube position should be to check the pH of stomach aspirate. If the pH is greater than 5.5, or obtaining aspirate is impossible, only then is an x-ray indicated for tube position checking. X-rays are easily misinterpreted, and exposing people to radiation unnecessarily is harmful. The implementation team conducted a theory-led audit to understand the extent of existing compliance with the guideline and the barriers and levers to developing practice and compliance. Using the Theoretical Domains Framework (TDF) (Atkins et al., 2017), they used a combination of surveys, an audit tool, and focus groups to understand the problem and design a change intervention that tackled the biggest barriers to the target behavior of checking pH as a first-line in NG tube placement. They then mapped barriers onto theoretically important domains from the TDF such as skills, beliefs about capabilities, and environmental context and resources. Using this map, they were able to design effective strategies for change. They used cues in the environment, for example, new care pathway documentation, to combat potential environmental contextual barriers/levers.

The results were statistically and clinically significant. They increased first-line pH use from 11% to 60%, decreased x-rays for placement from 60% to 37%, and reduced undocumented clinical practice around NG tube placement from 30% to 3% (Taylor et al., 2013). The estimated savings and costs in the first year were £2.56 million and £1.41 million respectively, giving a return on investment of 82%, projected to increase to 270% over 5 years (Taylor et al., 2014).

Theory helped the team make sense of complexity at diagnosis, planning, delivery, and evaluation stages of the improvement process. The qualitative comments contained in reflective logs of clinicians and interviews revealed that the process was feasible, was acceptable, and complemented rather than threatened local expertise.

CASE 4: PRIMARY CARE LEG ULCER CLINICS

A group of inner-city tissue viability nurse specialists (TVNs) wanted to tailor, implement. and audit their local guidelines on managing leg ulcers and then go on to set up two community-based leg ulcer clinics. The aim of this was to reduce variations in practice and outcomes across the organization and to reduce inappropriate referrals to an already busy complex wound clinic. We include this case study because although the entity of TVNs and leg ulcer clinics may be unique to some countries, the principles of the strategy adopted by the team are generalizable to change initiatives in other clinical settings.

The nurses developed a fivefold strategy:

- *Locally developed guidelines:* based on an inclusive, multidisciplinary development process that was actively "marketed" in trust settings at lunch times.
- *Opinion leaders:* the two well-respected TVNs worked with nurses, consultants, and local GPs.
- *Educational workshops:* these took place "in-service" and were aimed at familiarizing nurses with the guidelines and, crucially, learning to relate the guidelines to real patients and patient problems.
- *Targeted meetings and multidisciplinary training:* these focused on generating sufficient interest in practitioners so that they wanted to host clinics. The most enthusiastic practitioner in a local team was targeted with the intention that they would persuade their more skeptical colleagues.
- *Training and feedback:* the TVNs visited each clinic once a month and offered real-time training, support, and, crucially, the application of the guidelines during patient consultations.

This approach has led to the development of two clinics and a third in progress, with broad cross-disciplinary support for the new ways of working. However, the team failed to collect patient data before or after the development of the clinics, which meant they had no baseline criteria for measuring their success. As well as this design fault, the team had to struggle against the very real constraints of underfunding, recruitment difficulties, competing priorities, and variable morale and enthusiasm among staff.

The qualitative comments of staff indicate that small changes to the way clinical nurse specialists work (giving them a trustwide remit with responsibility for professional development) can yield good results, even in a less than perfect context: "Having (the nurse specialist) there to discuss different things makes a difference. When you are seeing seven leg ulcers in a row, it leads to better practice. We are using the leg ulcer care program lots …the professional development is the best part of it."

The team involved learned from their mistakes and tried to factor in solutions for the future: "We would invest a proportion of the project's resources in a baseline audit, because demonstrating improvement in healing rates provides the ultimate proof that an initiative to upgrade the care of patients with leg ulcers is working."

Ultimately, the researchers conclude that the team's greatest achievement was their contribution to the replacement of "…a severely fragmented, demoralized organization with one where staff are enthusiastic and open to learning." It seems that a very important "byproduct" of this initiative was the substantial cultural shift toward embracing learning and change.

CASE 5: KNOWLEDGE TO BEDSIDE CHANGE IMPLEMENTATION

This case demonstrates the evolution of an evidence-based culture over time. The Hospital Elder Life Program (HELP) is a model of care designed to prevent delirium and functional decline in hospitalized older persons (www.hospitalelderlifeprogram.org). The HELP model has its origins in a large prospective matched-control study of patients ($N = 852$) at risk for delirium (Inouye et al., 1999) that found patients experienced fewer numbers of days and less episodes of delirium upon receiving specialized care interventions.

HELP program interventions included: (i) daily visitation/orientation, (ii) sleep enhancement, (iii) oral volume repletion, (iv) feeding assistance, (v) mobilization, and (vi) hearing plus vision environmental adaptations. A dedicated team of geriatricians, nurse specialists, and trained volunteers delivered these interventions as a "bundle" aimed at preventing or mitigating complications germane to elderly people. More recently, additional bundle-based protocols aimed at prevention or mitigation of hypoxia, infection, constipation, and pain, have been developed (Yue et al., 2014). Notably, interventions tend to be non-pharmacological and require basic nursing care, for example, hand washing and mobilization. Evidence generated by Inouye et al. has informed clinical guidelines published by both the AHRQ (in the US) and NICE (in the UK) (Rubin et al., 2011).

Many organizations implement HELP to prevent delirium in geriatric patients (Rubin et al., 2011). Evaluations of implemented HELP programs report fewer iatrogenic complications, prevention of functional decline, and cost savings (Inouye et al. 1999, 2000, 2006, 2009; Rizzo et al., 2001). The scheme has spread beyond the US to Canada, the UK, Australia, and Taiwan (Bradley et al., 2006; Inouye et al., 2006).

Diffusing and sustaining evidence-based practice is challenging. In 2006, hospitals that contacted HELP ($N = 63$) were surveyed about how much of the HELP program they incorporated (Bradley et al., 2006). Twenty-five percent of respondents contracted with HELP for assistance with dissemination, 20.6% implemented programs similar to HELP, 20.6% reported adoption of HELP guidelines, and 33% did not implement any delirium prevention program. The most common reason was lack of senior management support, program expense, and lack of doctor and nurse dedication to the program.

In 2011, HELP transitioned to a web-based model. Before digitalization, transfer knowledge methods included publications, site visits, presentations at national conferences, publication, and grand rounds (Chen et al., 2015). Transition to a web-based platform provided broader reach and interactive consultation. Web users can access a program overview, training manuals, videos, and resources for professionals and carers. Telephone and e-mail support make the program easy to use and modify for local context with expert guidance from HELP.

In a survey of HELP website registrants ($N = 102$ sites), 39 (53%) implemented and maintained an active HELP model. Twenty-six (35%) sites used website resources to plan implementation, and 35 (50%) sites used the site to implement as well as support the program during and after launch. Forty-five sites (61%) used website resources for educational purposes, targeting healthcare professionals, patients, families, or volunteers. The digital version of HELP is a practical and innovative resource for knowledge transfer (Chen et al., 2015).

Studies of HELP program's diffusion describe the implementation of HELP in a community hospital setting (Rubin et al., 2011). As HELP was adopted between 2002 and 2008, delirium decreased by 15%, and patients were in hospital for almost 1 day less by 2008; costs avoided by preventing delirium was $7.3 m. These achievements were not without challenge. Staffing, teamwork, and monitoring barriers were overcome by strengthening the infrastructure, clarifying roles and responsibilities, focusing on recruitment and retention efforts, and maximizing routine electronic data collection. Sites that stayed closest to the HELP blueprint or model enjoyed the biggest benefits.

Conclusion: Culture, Practice Change, and Evidence-Based Health Care

There is a long established axiom that there are "no magic bullets" (Oxman et al., 1995) to implement new knowledge and innovation required for evidence-based change. But with the help of appropriate theoretical frameworks, you can give yourself and your team a fighting chance of successfully introducing changes.

Practically, the clinician or manager considering change should employ a good diagnostic workup of the factors likely to hinder or promote research use in decisions. This should focus on the levels of individuals, teams, and the organization and consider strategically targeting barriers and subgroups within each of these elements. Moreover, initial efforts should focus on those areas over which the team has some control (e.g., the roles of key individuals such as the clinical nurse specialist or the link nurse; and the support and nature of information technology and skills training). It has been said there is nothing more practical than a good theory (Eysenck, 1987); when it comes to changing cultures for evidence based practice, never has it been truer.

References

American Nurses Association, 2015. Nursing: Scope and Standards of Practice, third ed. American Nurses Association, Inc. Publications. Silver Spring, Maryland.

Allen, D., Gillen, E., Rixson, L., 2009. The effectiveness of integrated care pathways for adults and children in health care settings: a systematic review. JBI. Libr. Syst. Rev. 7 (3), 80–129.

Ashburner, L., 2001. Organisational Behaviour and Organisation Studies in Health Care: Reflections on the Future. Palgrave, Basingstoke, UK.

Atkins, L., Francis, J., Islam, R., et al., 2017. A guide to using the Theoretical Domains Framework of behaviour change to investigate implementation problems. Implement. Sci. 12 (1), 77.

Black, A.T., Balneaves, L.G., Garossino, C., Puyat, J.H., Qian, H., 2015. Promoting evidence-based practice through a research training program for point-of-care clinicians. J. Nurs. Adm. 45 (1), 14–20.

Bradley, E.H., Webster, T.R., Schlesinger, M., Baker, D., Inouye, S.K., 2006. Patterns of diffusion of evidence-based clinical programmes: a case study of the Hospital Elder Life Program. Qual. Saf. Health Care 15 (5), 334–338.

Braithwaite, J., Churruca, K., Ellis, L.A., et al., 2017. Complexity science in healthcare—aspirations, approaches, applications and accomplishments: A white paper. Australian Institute of Health Innovation and Macquarie University, New South Wales, Australia.

Brody, A.A., Barnes, K., Ruble, C., Sakowski, J., 2012. Evidence-based practice councils: potential path to staff nurse empowerment and leadership growth. J. Nurs. Adm. 42 (1), 28–33.

Cadmus, E., Van Wynen, E.A., Chamberlain, B., et al., 2008. Nurses' skill level and access to evidence-based practice. J. Nurs. Adm. 38 (11), 494–503.

Cameron, G., Wren, A.M., 1999. Reconstructing organizational culture: a process using multiple perspectives. Public Health Nurs. 16 (2), 96–101.

Canadian Nurses Association, 2017. Code of Ethics for Registered Nurses. ISBN: 978-1-55119-441-7. Available from: www.cna-aiic.ca. Accessed 14.06.18.

Chaillet, N., Dube, E., Dugas, M., et al., 2006. Evidence-based strategies for implementing guidelines in obstetrics: a systematic review. Obstet. Gynecol. 108 (5), 1234–1245.

Chassin, M.R., Loeb, J.M., 2013. High-reliability health care: getting there from here. Milbank Q. 91 (3), 459–490.

Chassin, M.R., Loeb, J.M., Schmaltz, S.P., Wachter, R.M., 2010. Accountability measures—using measurement to promote quality improvement. N. Engl. J. Med. 363 (7), 683–688.

Chen, P., Dowal, S., Schmitt, E., et al., 2015. Hospital Elder Life Program in the real world: the many uses of the Hospital Elder Life Program website. J. Am. Geriatr. Soc. 63 (4), 797–803.

Davies, H.T., Nutley, S.M., Mannion, R., 2000. Organisational culture and quality of health care. Qual. Health Care 9 (2), 111–119.

Denis, J.L., Lehoux, P., 2013. Organizational theories. In: Straus, S.E., Tetroe, M.A., Graham, I.D. (Eds.), Knowledge Translation in Healthcare: Moving from Evidence to Practice. John Wiley & Sons, London, pp. 308–319.

Department of Health and Social Care, 2010. Essence of Care 2010. Gateway Ref:14641. Available from: https://www.gov.uk/government/publications/essence-of-care-2010. Accessed 20.04.19.

Eppler, M.J., Mengis, J., 2009. How communicators can fight information overload. Comm.World 42 (1), 28–33.

Estabrooks, C.A., Squires, J.E., Cummings, G.G., Birdsell, J.M., Norton, P.G., 2009. Development and assessment of the Alberta Context Tool. BMC Health Serv. Res. 9, 234.

Eysenck, H.J., 1987. There is nothing more practical than a good theory (Kurt Lewin)—true or false? Adv. Psychol. 40, 49–64.

Forsetlund, L., Bjorndal, A., Rashidian, A., et al., 2009. Continuing education meetings and workshops: effects on professional practice and health care outcomes. Cochrane Database Syst. Rev. (2), CD003030.

Muir Gray, J.A., 1997. Evidence-Based Healthcare: How to Make Health Policy and Management Decisions. Churchill Livingstone, London.

Graystone, R., 2017. The 2019 Magnet Application Manual: nursing excellence standards evolving with practice. J. Nurs. Adm. 47 (11), 527–528.

Greenhalgh, T., Robert, G., Bate, P., Kyriakidou, O., Macfarlane, F., Peacock, R., 2005. Diffusion of Innovations in Health Service Organisations: A Systematic Literature Review. Blackwell, Oxford.

Helfrich, C.D., Li, Y.F., Sharp, N.D., Sales, A.E., 2009. Organizational readiness to change assessment (ORCA), development of an instrument based on the Promoting Action on Research in Health Services (PARIHS) framework. Implement. Sci. 4, 38.

Iles, V., Sutherland, K., 2001. Organisational change: a review for health care managers, professionals and researchers. Service Delivery and Organisation Research and Development Programme. National Co-ordinating Centre for Service Delivery and Organisation R&D, London.

Inouye, S.K., Baker, D.I., Fugal, P., Bradley, E.H., Project, H.D., 2006. Dissemination of the hospital elder life program: implementation, adaptation, and successes. J. Am. Geriatr. Soc. 54 (10), 1492–1499.

Inouye, S.K., Bogardus Jr., S.T., Baker, D.I., Leo-Summers, L., Cooney Jr., L.M., 2000. The Hospital Elder Life Program: a model of care to prevent cognitive and functional decline in older hospitalized patients. Hospital Elder Life Program. J. Am. Geriatr. Soc. 48 (12), 1697–1706.

Inouye, S.K., Bogardus Jr., S.T., Charpentier, P.A., Leo-Summers, L., Acampora, D., Holford, T.R., et al., 1999. A multicomponent intervention to prevent delirium in hospitalized older patients. N. Engl. J. Med. 340 (9), 669–676.

Inouye, S.K., Brown, C.J., Tinetti, M.E., 2009. Medicare nonpayment, hospital falls, and unintended consequences. N. Engl. J. Med. 360 (23), 2390–2393.

Institute of Medicine (US), 2000. Committee on Quality of Health Care in America. In: Kohn, L.T., Corrigan, J.M., Donaldson, M.S. (Eds.), To err is human: Building a safer health system. National Academies Press, Washington, DC.

Institute of Medicine, 2010. Redesigning the clinical effectiveness research paradigm: innovation and practice-based approaches: Workshop summary. National Academies Press, Washington, DC.

Johnson, M.J., May, C.R., 2015. Promoting professional behaviour change in healthcare: what interventions work, and why? A theory-led overview of systematic reviews. BMJ Open 5 (9), e008592.

Kash, B.A., Spaulding, A., Gamm, L., Johnson, C.E., 2013. Health care administrators' perspectives on the role of absorptive capacity for strategic change initiatives: a qualitative study. Health Care Manag. Rev. 38 (4), 339–348.

Kavanagh, M.H., Ashkanasy, N.M., 2006. The impact of leadership and change management strategy on organizational culture and individual acceptance of change during a merger. Br. J. Manag. 17, S81–S103.

Kimber, M., Barwick, M., Fearing, G., 2012. Becoming an evidence-based service provider: staff perceptions and experiences of organizational change. J. Behav. Health Serv. Res. 39 (3), 314–332.

Lawton, R.E., Armitage, G.E., 2012. Innovating for Patient Safety in Medicine. Sage Publications, London.

Mannion, R., Smith, J., 2018. Hospital culture and clinical performance: where next? BMJ Quality Saf. 27 (3), 179–181.

May, C., Finch, T., Mair, F., et al., 2007. Understanding the implementation of complex interventions in health care: the normalization process model. BMC Health Serv. Res. 7, 148.

May, C.R., Mair, F., Finch, T., et al., 2009. Development of a theory of implementation and integration: Normalization Process Theory. Implement. Sci. 4, 29.

May, C., Rapley, T., Mair, F.S., et al., 2015. Normalization Process Theory On-line Users' Manual, Toolkit and NoMAD instrument. Available from: http://www.normalizationprocess.org. Accessed 20.04.19.

McCormack, B., McCarthy, G., Wright, J., Slater, P., Coffey, A., 2009. Development and testing of the Context Assessment Index (CAI). Worldviews Evid. Based Nurs. 6 (1), 27–35.

McLaughlin, M.K., Gabel Speroni, K., Kelly, K.P., Guzzetta, C.E., Desale, S., 2013. National survey of hospital nursing research, part 1: research requirements and outcomes. J. Nurs. Adm. 43 (1), 10–17.

Newhouse, R.P., 2010. Instruments to assess organizational readiness for evidence-based practice. J. Nurs. Adm. 40 (10), 404–407.

National Health Service England, 2017. NHS England Research Plan. NHS England, London.

Nursing and Midwifery Council, 2018. The Code: Professional Standards of Practice and Behaviour for Nurses and Midwives. Nursing and Midwifery Council, London.

Nursing Council of New Zealand, 2012. Code of Conduct for Nurses. ISBN: 978-0-908662-45-6. Available from: www.nursingcouncil.org.nz. Accessed 14.06.18.

Nursing and Midwifery Board of Australia, 2016. Registered Nurse Standards for Practice. Available from: http://www.nursingmidwiferyboard.gov.au/Codes-Guidelines-Statements/Professional-standards/registered-nurse-standards-for-practice.aspx. Accessed 14.06.18.

Oxman, A.D., Thomson, M.A., Davis, D.A., Haynes, R.B., 1995. No magic bullets—a systematic review of 102 trials of interventions to improve professional practice. CMAJ 153 (10), 1423–1431.

Page, A., 2004. Keeping Patients Safe: Transforming the Work Environment of Nurses. National Academies Press, Washington, DC.

Resar, R., Pronovost, P., Haraden, C., Simmonds, T., Rainey, T., Nolan, T., 2005. Using a bundle approach to improve ventilator care processes and reduce ventilator-associated pneumonia. Jt. Comm. J. Qual. Patient Saf. 31 (5), 243–248.

Rizzo, J.A., Bogardus Jr., S.T., Leo-Summers, L., Williams, C.S., Acampora, D., Inouye, S.K., 2001. Multicomponent targeted intervention to prevent delirium in hospitalized older patients: what is the economic value? Med. Care 39 (7), 740–752.

Rubin, F.H., Neal, K., Fenlon, K., Hassan, S., Inouye, S.K., 2011. Sustainability and scalability of the hospital elder life program at a community hospital. J. Am. Geriatr. Soc. 59 (2), 359–365.

Sales, A., Lurie, N., Moscovice, I., Goes, J., 1995. Is quality in the eye of the beholder? Jt. Comm. J. Qual. Improv. 21 (5), 219–225.

Sales, A.E., 2013. Reflections on the state of nursing implementation science. Int. J. Nurs. Stud. 50 (4), 443–444.

Schön, D.A., 1994. The reflective practitioner: how professionals think in action. Routledge, Taylor and Francis Group, London and New York.

Seidl, K.L., Newhouse, R.P., 2012. The intersection of evidence-based practice with 5 quality improvement methodologies. J. Nurs. Admin. 42 (6), 299–304.

Taylor, N., Lawton, R., Moore, S., et al., 2014. Collaborating with front-line healthcare professionals: the clinical and cost effectiveness of a theory based approach to the implementation of a national guideline. BMC Health Serv. Res. 14, 648.

Taylor, N., Lawton, R., Slater, B., Foy, R., 2013. The demonstration of a theory-based approach to the design of localized patient safety interventions. Implement. Sci. 8, 123.

Thompson, C., Pulleyblank, R., Parrott, S., Essex, H., 2016. The cost-effectiveness of quality improvement projects: a conceptual framework, checklist and online tool for considering the costs and consequences of implementation-based quality improvement. J. Eval. Clin. Pract. 22 (1), 26–30.

Weeks, S.M., Moore, P., Allender, M., 2011. A regional evidence-based practice fellowship: collaborating competitors. J. Nurs. Adm. 41 (1), 10–14.

Yue, J., Tabloski, P., Dowal, S.L., Puelle, M.R., Nandan, R., Inouye, S.K., 2014. NICE to HELP: operationalizing National Institute for Health and Clinical Excellence guidelines to improve clinical practice. J. Am. Geriatr. Soc. 62 (4), 754–761.

Zhang, A.Y., Tsui, A.S., Song, L.J., Li, C., Jia, L., 2008. How do I trust thee? The employee–organization relationship, supervisory support, and middle manager trust in the organization. Hum. Res. Manag. 47 (11), 111–132.

Absolute risk reduction (ARR) and increase (ARI): The size of the difference between outcomes in the intervention (or exposure) group and outcomes in the control group. It is the absolute arithmetical difference between the experimental (or exposure) event rate (EER) and the control event rate (CER). To calculate: [EER – CER].

Action research: Investigators and participants collaborate to improve a social situation through change interventions. The emphasis is on professional development and empowerment of participants.

Allocation concealment: Ensuring that the person who enrolls an individual into a study is unaware of the group to which that individual will be allocated. Techniques include using sequentially numbered, sealed, opaque envelopes, with each envelope containing details of the group to which that individual is to be allocated (e.g., group A or group B). Central randomization services are also used, in which people not involved in the study hold the randomization details. At the time of allocating the individual to a group, the investigator contacts the service (this may be an online, automated service) to find out whether that individual is to go into group A or group B.

Bias: Systematic error in the design, conduct, or interpretation of a study that may distort the results of the study away from the "truth."

Blinding (masking): Concealing whether or not the participant is receiving (or has received) the experimental intervention. In an ideal study, the research participants, the people administering the intervention(s), the people assessing the outcomes, and the data analysts will be blinded. The terms *single-blind*, *double-blind*, or *triple-blind* are sometimes used to indicate the level of blinding. For example, when both the participants and the investigators assessing the outcomes are blinded, the trial may be classified as double-blind. However, it is important to note that these terms are not used consistently. Also, it is not possible to guess from the terms themselves which groups were blinded.

Boolean operators: Used when searching electronic databases to combine search terms. They include AND, OR, and NOT.

Case control study: An observational study in which a group of individuals with the target disorder (cases) and a group of individuals without the target disorder (controls) are identified. Researchers look back in time to try and identify whether the exposure of interest was more prevalent in one group than the other.

Case series: A study reporting on a series of patients who have all experienced an outcome of interest, and in which there is no control group.

Case study: An in-depth investigation of an individual person, group of people, organization, or event using a variety of sources of data.

CATs and CATmaker software: CAT is the abbreviated term for critically appraised topic. It is a summary of individual item(s) of evidence created in response to an information need. The Centre for Evidence-Based Medicine produces *CATmaker* software that can be used to create CATs and includes a facility to calculate figures, such as the number needed to treat and so on.

Clinical effectiveness: This term is used in two ways. First, it is used as shorthand for the processes used to improve the quality of health care. Second, it is used to refer to the extent to which a specific clinical intervention, when deployed in the field for a particular patient or population, delivers the intended outcomes such that the benefits outweigh the harms.

Clinical governance: A framework through which healthcare organizations are accountable for continuously improving the quality of health services and safeguarding high standards of care.

Cohort study: An observational study in which patients exposed to a drug or other agent are identified and followed forward in time to see whether they develop particular outcomes. People not exposed to the agent (i.e., a control group) may be included in the study.

Confidence interval (CI): Research studies use samples from the population. If the same study was carried out 100 times on different samples of the same population, 100 different results would be obtained. These results would spread around a true but unknown value. The confidence interval estimates this sampling variation. Thus we can think of the confidence interval as the range within which it is probable that the population value lies. It is possible to calculate this range from the data obtained in a single study. By convention, the 95% confidence interval is often used, that is, the true population value will lie between the specified range in 95% of cases. For example, if a study reported a difference in mortality rates between two groups as 10% with an upper 95% CI limit of 13% and a lower 95% confidence limit of 7%, we know that in 95% of cases the true mortality difference for the population is between 7% and 13%.

Confirmability: The extent to which research findings are determined by participants rather than by the perspectives or motives of the researcher.

Confounder: A factor that affects the observed relationship between the variables under investigation.

Constant comparative analysis: Used in qualitative studies, the researcher constantly seeks out cases in the data set during the collection of the data that support or "shape" provisional hypotheses.

Control event rate (CER): This is the proportion of individuals in the control group in whom the outcome (event) is observed.

Control group: The control group in a study is that group of individuals who do not receive the intervention or exposure, or who receive a placebo. Their outcomes are compared with those of the intervention group (the group receiving the intervention or exposure). They serve to "control" for whether the patients in the intervention group would have improved or deteriorated regardless of the intervention or exposure.

Convergent parallel: A study design used in mixed methods research, in which both quantitative and qualitative elements of the study are conducted separately in parallel and integrated at the stage of analysis.

Credibility: The extent to which findings are believable.

Critical appraisal: The process of systematically evaluating a piece of evidence in terms of validity (i.e., the extent to which the results may be affected by bias), findings (i.e., interpreting the results), and applicability (i.e., the extent to which the findings may be applicable to your own clinical setting/patients).

Cross-sectional study: Data are collected from a representative sample of individuals at the same point in time.

Dependability: Used in qualitative research, the extent to which research findings are repeatable if the research is repeated in the same or similar participants or context.

Ethnography: The nature of organizations, culture, or communities in their native settings.

Experimental event rate (EER): The proportion of participants in the treatment (intervention) group in whom the outcome (event) is observed.

Explanatory sequential: A study design used in mixed methods research in which the quantitative study is undertaken and analyzed first, followed by a qualitative study that explains the quantitative results in more depth.

Exploratory sequential: A study design used in mixed methods research in which the initial study is qualitative with the results used to inform and develop a second quantitative study.

Grounded theory: Development of new theoretical perspectives based on (grounded in) individuals' lived experiences.

Incidence: The number of new cases of a disease occurring during a specified period in the population at risk.

Intention-to-treat analysis: Study participants are analyzed in the groups to which they were randomized, even if they did not receive the planned intervention or if they deviated from the study protocol. Intention-to-treat analysis mimics real-life situations because it investigates the outcomes after a management decision to use a particular treatment.

Inter-rater (or inter-observer) reliability: Measures the extent to which an instrument or test gives consistent results when applied by different investigators under exactly the same circumstances and where the variable being measured remains unchanged.

Intra-rater (or intra-observer) reliability: Measures the extent to which an instrument or test gives consistent results when applied by the same investigator at two or more time points under exactly the same circumstances and where the variable being measured remains unchanged.

Kappa coefficient (κ): A statistical test used to indicate the extent of agreement between observers' measurements, adjusted for the amount of agreement that could be expected due to chance alone. The results are reported between 0 and 1. The nearer the result is to 1, the better the agreement between the observers' measurements.

Likelihood ratio: See **negative likelihood ratio** and **positive likelihood ratio.**

Median: The midpoint on a scale. One-half of the observations have a value less than or equal to the median, and one-half have a value greater than or equal to the median.

Member (respondent) checking: Used in qualitative research, the process of feeding back the researcher's interpretations of the data to informants (the people involved in generating the data) to determine whether they recognize and agree with them.

Meta-analysis: Used in systematic reviews, this is the process of statistically combining the (quantitative) results from a number of studies. It should only be used to combine quantitative results if appropriate.

Meta-synthesis: Used in systematic reviews, this is the interpretive integration of findings from a number of qualitative studies.

Mixed methods research (MMR): A research approach that encompasses both quantitative and qualitative research methods in a single study or program of enquiry, designed to address research questions or phenomena that cannot be answered by only using quantitative or qualitative methods.

Narrative enquiry: Exploring the lives of individuals through their narratives or stories.

Naturalistic enquiry: Relating to qualitative research, phenomena are studied within their natural setting rather than within a superficial or controlled one. The approach aims to minimize investigator manipulation of the study setting and places no prior constraint on what the outcomes will be.

Negative case analysis: Used in qualitative research, the process of actively searching for cases that appear to be inconsistent with the emerging analysis.

Negative likelihood ratio: The ratio of true-negative results to false-negative results. A negative likelihood ratio of 0.5 means that a negative test result is one-half as likely to occur in patients with the condition as in patients without the condition.

Negative predictive value: The proportion of people with negative test results who do not have the target disorder (should be high).

Number needed to harm: The number of patients to receive the intervention for one additional person to experience an episode of harm, over a specified period. To calculate: 1/ARR.

Number needed to treat: The number of patients that need to be treated if a beneficial outcome is to occur in one additional person. To calculate: 1/ARR.

Odds: The probability of an event happening, that is, the ratio of the number of people having the outcome of interest to the number of people not having the outcome of interest.

Odds ratio: The ratio of the odds of an event in the treatment (or exposure) group compared with the odds of the event in the control (or unexposed) group.

Ontology: Relates to the nature of things within the world: the assumptions and beliefs we hold about how the world is made up.

PECOS: A question framework for building focused questions, in particular questions about the effects of exposure on a health outcome. The letters denote *P*opulation, *E*xposure, *C*omparison (usually no exposure), *O*utcome, and *S*tudy design.

Phenomenology: Relates to the nature of individuals' personal experiences.

PICOS: A question framework for building focused questions, in particular questions about the effects of an intervention or therapy. The letters denote *P*opulation, *I*ntervention, *C*omparison intervention, *O*utcome, and *S*tudy design.

Placebo: In the context of a placebo-controlled clinical trial, a biologically inert substance given to participants in the control arm of a trial. The placebo is similar in every other way to the biologically active intervention administered to participants in the treatment arm of the trial. It is used to conceal which arm of the trial the participants are in.

Positive likelihood ratio: The ratio of true-positive results to false-positive results. A positive likelihood ratio of 8.5 means that a positive test result is 8.5 times as likely to occur in patients with the condition as in patients without the condition. (A positive likelihood ratio of 1 means that a positive test is equally as likely to occur in patients with the condition as in patients without the condition.)

Positive predictive value: The proportion of people with positive test results who have the target disorder (should be high).

Pragmatism: The underlying philosophy underpinning mixed methods research studies, which focuses on "what works."

Prevalence: This is the number of cases or events (e.g., measles, smokers) in a defined population at a given point in time.

Process evaluation: Often running in parallel with a randomized controlled trial, process evaluations can be used to understand how an intervention works and in what context. They typically use mixed methods as the basis for the evaluation.

Qualitative research: Seeks to describe phenomena through the meanings, experiences, practices, and views of individuals within their natural settings. Qualitative research aims to understand real-world situations as they unfold, from the point of view of the people who live in these worlds.

Quantitative research: Seeks to describe phenomena through measuring and quantifying the relationship between the variables or characteristics being studied.

Random allocation: Individuals participating in the trial have a defined probability (usually 50%, i.e., an equal chance) of being allocated to either the intervention or the control group. Computer packages or printed random number tables are usually used to generate a list of random numbers (i.e., numbers with no discernable sequence or order) that indicate the group to which each individual is to be randomized. So, for example, even numbers might indicate allocation to the intervention group and odd numbers to the control group. The group to which each individual is to be allocated is not predictable.

Randomized controlled trial (RCT): A study in which individuals are assigned to the experimental intervention group or to the comparison group(s) by random allocation.

Reflexivity: A technique used in qualitative research, especially in the analysis of data, where the author reflects on how she or he may have shaped or influenced the research findings.

Relative benefit increase (RBI): The proportional increase in rates of beneficial events between the experimental and control groups. To calculate: [EER − CER]/CER.

Relative risk (RR): The ratio of the risk in one group compared with the other.

Relative risk increase (RRI): The proportional increase in rates of harmful or undesirable events between the experimental and control groups. To calculate: [EER − CER]/CER.

Relative risk reduction (RRR): The proportional reduction in rates of harmful or undesirable events between the experimental and control groups. To calculate: [EER − CER]/CER.

Reliability: See inter-rater and intra-rater reliability.

Sample: Research is carried out on a subgroup of the population. This subgroup is often referred to as the study sample. A variety of sampling methods can be employed to select the sample depending on the purpose of the research.

Sampling: The process by which a subset of the (target) population is selected.

Sensitivity: When applied to diagnostic tests, sensitivity refers to the proportion of people with a target disorder who have a positive test result.

Specificity: When applied to diagnostic tests, specificity refers to the proportion of people who do not have a target disorder who have a negative test result.

SPICE: A question framework for building focused questions about people's perspectives, decisions, behaviors, or experiences. The letters denote *S*etting, *P*erspective, *I*nterest (Phenomenon of), *C*omparison, and *E*valuation.

Statistical significance: The likelihood of a result occurring by chance. By convention, the level at which a result is said to be statistically significant is set at 5%, that is, when there is a less than 5% probability that the result happened by chance, it is said to be statistically significant. This is usually written in the form of $p < 0.05$. The p-value does not, however, tell us how clinically important the result is.

Systematic review: A summary of research evidence pertinent to a specified question in which systematic and explicit methods are used to identify, select, critically appraise, and synthesize the available research evidence. Systematic reviews are research studies in their own right and are sometimes called "secondary research."

Thick description: A term used in qualitative research. A very detailed account of the methodological and interpretive strategy in the form of field notes.

Transferability: The extent to which research findings are transferable from the context within which the research study was undertaken to another context.

Triangulation: The phenomenon under investigation is examined from different perspectives using two or more methods (or data sources/theories/investigators). Findings of the different methods are cross-checked and interpreted against each other.

Truncation: Used in searching electronic databases, truncation ensures that all terms that have the same text stem are found. For example, a search for the truncated word "child" will retrieve articles containing the terms "child," "childhood," "childless," "children," and so on. The truncation symbol varies according to the database provider. Examples of symbols are the asterisk (child*), dollar sign (child$), or % sign (child%).

Wildcard: Used in searching electronic databases, a wildcard is a character (in some databases it is a ?) that can be used to replace one or more characters within a word so that articles will be retrieved regardless of the way in which the word is spelled. For example, if the term "p?ediatric" is searched, articles using the American spelling (pediatric) and articles using the British spelling (paediatric) will be retrieved.

INDEX

Note: Page numbers followed by "f" indicate figures and "t" indicate tables.